GROWING STRAIGHT

A NEW SYSTEM OF PHYSICAL EDUCATION

with

MENTAL CONTROL

BY

MAUD SMITH WILLIAMS

AS PRACTICED BY
THE NORTH AMERICAN INDIANS

Illustrated by
THE AUTHOR

Maud Smith Williams

NEWCASTLE PUBLISHING CO. INC.
NORTH HOLLYWOOD, CALIFORNIA
1981

A NEWCASTLE BOOK
FIRST PRINTING OCTOBER 1981
PRINTED IN THE UNITED STATES OF AMERICA

CONTENTS

PART I

FOREWORD

Something New

The youth of the Twentieth Century complain that the old methods of living are out of date for them! Further, they demand a physical training with mental and emotional control; something adequate to meet their needs of today and to prepare them for the future. Zenophon tells us that the best man is always studying how to improve, and that he is happiest who feels he is improving; American educators are ever seeking improvement in both mental and physical educational systems.

G. Stanley Hall, in his remarkable work, "Youth, its Education, Regimen, and Hygiene," points out the need of something *different,* yet combining the best in the different schools of athletics; also, that the danger of our present systems lies in their *inflexibility* and over-scholastic treatment, advising the need of a great range of variations, if it would do more. He favors what the Indian has long known, that "in the very act of *stretching,* for which much is to be said, *Nature itself suggests correctives and preventives."*

It is true, as he states, that our ideals, while closely related, are as yet far from harmonized. Swedish, Turner, Sargent, and American systems are each, most unfortunately, still too blind to the others' merits and too conscious of the others' shortcomings. To the same extent they are, by narrow devotion to a single cult, prevented from getting together. This inability of leaders to combine causes uncertainty and lack of confidence in, and of enthusiastic support for, any system on the part of the public. And here Prof. Hall puts in a strong plea for the need of a *new system* by a *different person* with *different ideals and with the addition of both mental and psychic (soul) culture.*

After studying every known system of physical education to date and carefully extracting the essence of their benefits, the author came to the conclusion, as did Prof. Hall, that there was something decidedly lacking. That lack is supplied by the American Indian; he has been in possession of this precious knowledge for ages.

Few persons care to emulate Hercules. An overdevelopment of muscles is neither satisfactory nor useful to modern civilization. Furthermore, unless strenuous exercise is kept up continuously, the athlete becomes muscle-bound, sick, or fat. "We do not want 'will-virtuosos,' who perform feats hard to learn, but easy to do and good for show; nor spurtiness of any sort which develops an erethic habit of work, temper, and circulation, and is favored by some of our popular sports, but too soon reacts into fatigue. The trouble is that few realize what vigor is in man or woman, or how endurance and self-control, no less than great achievement, *depend on muscle habits.*"

And here is where the Indian's system excels. Muscle habits are formed through the power of mind. By employing the will in every action while at the same time developing self-control, one gains endurance and the power to achieve.

The New Age

We are facing the dawn of a new era, an age when right will supersede might. A new light already casts its glow over the horizon and the bugle calls the wise to prepare. The brilliant young people of this new generation need all the coöperation of will power, self-control and diplomacy of which their minds and bodies are capable in order to meet the demands of their future. They face an era of arbitration, of reason, of clever mind pitted against clever mind.

The best body implies the best mind. The Greeks could hardly conceive bodily, apart from psychic (soul), education, and physical development was for the sake of mental training. They further held that if physical perfection was cultivated, moral and mental excellence would follow, and that without this, national culture rests on an insecure basis. One-half of all education was devoted to the body. Galton says the Greeks excelled us as much as we do the African negro. In our day there are many new reasons to believe that the best nations of the future will be those which give most intelligent care to the body. To acquire the power of doing all with full consciousness and with volition, *mentalizes the body,* gives control over the higher brain levels and develops them by rescuing activities from the dominance of the lower centers and emotional impulses.

Assuredly, the ideal human being should be developed evenly, on all planes of normal activity, *physical, mental* and *spiritual,* at one and the same time.

Perfect alignment of the spine and the major nerve centers with the head and neck are absolutely requisite for efficient brain service.

Equipoise of body with the development of will power and clear thinking are as essential to mental progress as a healthy brain and nervous system are to perfect kinesthetic control.

The American Indian has preserved secrets of physical and mental development from a past civilization that is said to be superior to anything we know today. It is fitting at this time that an important part of this valuable knowledge should come to light and be preserved to humanity for all time.

CHAPTER I

HOW THE INDIAN'S SYSTEM IS DIFFERENT

This method of body building and corrective physical training has been developed through intimate contact with American Indians of many tribes. It is founded upon the secret knowledge of old Indian adepts and true Medicine men, having been handed down from generation to generation by word of mouth. These teachers instructed their people to develop *body, mind and soul together,* in accordance with Nature's laws, laws which they had penetrated deeply. Only to one who has studied the red man's methods and has learned for himself the carefully concealed knowledge does he admit the facts, and then only after the discoverer has proven himself a worthy and trusted friend. The author has worked long and earnestly to learn the Indian's method, and, while giving him full credit for its conception, believes this is the first attempt to present it to the young people of our day in a scientific system of physical education and one which meets with their desires for something new, inclusive and different.

Simple

Simplicity is the keynote of the entire work. Long words and technical terms have been carefully avoided. Simple language is used throughout, making it easy for anyone to understand. The Indian system is easy to learn and easy to do ; anyone can master it. Full directions accompany the exercises with broken-line illustrations, the heavier lines showing the weight placement and the muscles used in the movements, and the light lines indicating the muscles kept flexible or relaxed.

Natural and Normal

First and foremost the Indian system of physical education is something more than mere athletics. The Indians believe, as did the Greeks and Oriental peoples, that a normal physical training must include, at the same time, both mental and ethical training. Each naturally compliments the other, since man is essentially triune in his nature, having a body, mind and soul ; each part of him depends more or less upon the other parts for complete expression. Therefore, this is not merely

I

a book of physical exercises but a guide, at the same time, to mental and emotional control.

The principles as well as the methods of this system form a foundation work for all forms of physical education, physical training and corrective therapeutics. The work is in no way restricted to short period exercises, but may be incorporated into all sorts of motions, at work, exercise, or play. The Indian's method of weight-placement and movement, with its mental and muscular control, may be literally lived every hour of the day, continuously, in every act and motion, and is a constant source of benefit. It is obvious that exercises which may be practiced in every circumstance of life and at all times, whatever the occupation, are of far greater value than those used only occasionally. Being much broader in scope than mere athletic training it is infinitely more interesting. It is neither mechanical nor monotonous, and, being perfectly natural, it produces normality while developing the individual through natural, sensible and practical methods.

Psychological

Because of its deep psychological effects, its mental control, its ethical and æsthetic culture, this system is unique and meets with the instant approval of all interested in higher education as well as those who appreciate the enormous value of combining mental with physical training.

Since thoughts of some sort are constantly running through the mind, anyway, we believe it is far more beneficial to direct constructive thoughts into proper channels while exercising, thus gradually gaining absolute control over the body as well as the mind and emotions. This is a tremendous aid in developing will power as well as in controlling the desires and impulses; it gradually mentalizes the body while developing great strength and endurance, and, at the same time, keeping one healthy and happy.

The kind and quality of thoughts employed while using a certain set of muscles have a direct bearing upon the *kind of power generated in the body*. This combination is very effective in its subtlety, producing the most amazing and satisfactory results quite simply.

Methods

The outstanding feature of "Growing Straight" lies in how the work is done. While many of the exercises given herein may seem familiar, in reality they are quite different from other systems. We are naturally limited to three sets of motions, to and from the body, and rotary. But the manner in which the muscles are used is different and the posture while exercising is different, while the thoughts and will power, being definitely directionalized, produce very definite results. Furthermore, the entire system is based upon flexibility rather than upon tension or rigidity; upon periods of relaxation following all contractions and upon rhythms of motion. Particular attention is given to rhythmic breathing, the cultivation of grace and poise, the alignment of the head and spine, and the proper placement of the internal organs. The whole secret lies in *how* you work and how you *think while you work*. Preference is always given the *method of procedure* over the number of times a motion is made or the speed with which it is executed. Speed is as much a matter of flexibility and habit as strength is the result of growth.

Dramatic Appeal

With its strong dramatic appeal the Indian system is at once attractive to both young and old. We are all eager to acquire a knowledge heretofore held secret and mysterious. It is a powerful, graceful, colorful method of education, filled with hidden meanings and capable of easy receptivity. It awakens a deep appreciation of Nature together with an underlying feeling of joy and happiness.

For Everyone

The business man, the laborer, the housewife, the college student, the child, and even the invalid, as well as those leading a sedentary life, will find that by incorporating the principles of the Indian's system into their lives they will be enormously benefited, their health assured and their lives lengthened.

Outdoor Sports

—such as tennis, riding, swimming, walking, bowling, football, baseball, polo, may all be practiced to much greater advantage under this system, for it is invaluable in limbering up the joints or muscles and in building up great strength and endurance.

Dancers

—acrobats and entertainers can double their ability and greatly enhance their resistance and endurance while lengthening their lives and the period of their usefulness by employing these principles in their own line of work.

Golf

Devotees of the grand old Scotch game will find herein that ability to relax and become perfectly flexible so heartily extolled by all professionals. One may acquire an easy, graceful and forceful swing without that "tightening up" or nerve tension. Mental hazards are easily overcome, along with that depression following poor shots. Your game will improve fifty per cent and your strength and endurance will treble.

What It Will Do for You

This system will absolutely remodel the entire body, producing a more perfect symmetry of form. At the same time it will produce rugged endurance and subtle strength, with graceful movement and poise.

It is conducive to health, strength and longevity.

It develops will power and conquers emotional impulses.

It develops brain power and gives mental control.

It teaches alertness, quickness of thought and action, and trains the mind to concentrate, therefore producing greater efficiency.

It teaches the art of relaxation so much needed in this strenuous age. Flexibility of body and mind are basic principles for any kind of growth.

It teaches how to obtain absolute freedom from all nervous tension.

It stimulates the circulation of the blood and nerve currents.

It relieves undue pressure upon the vital organs and all strain upon the muscles, nerves and feet.

It relieves the spine of all strain, retaining the supple litheness of youth.

It develops a graceful contour, remarkable strength, and great endurance. One becomes practically tireless.

The muscles acquire a catlike grace along with great agility and swiftness of movement.

It is very effective in stimulating and regulating glandular function, and, in conjunction with proper sun and water baths and diet, is a preventive against disease.

The Indian has learned the secret of keeping fit. He knows how to speed up resistance, how to create energy within himself, and how to overcome any tendency to laziness or weariness. His endurance is notorious.

If you are underweight the Indian system will build you up.

If you are overweight the Indian system will reduce you.

SEVEN RULES OF LIFE

1. Correct Posture and Carriage

Both posture and carriage are so essential to good health that their importance can hardly be overestimated. Success in business as well as in social life depends much upon personal appearance. A good posture is an aid to self-confidence; a good carriage demands somewhat of deference and respect from others. Both are cultivated along with balance and poise through physical training with *mental control*. Persistent effort, while employing the basic principles of the Indian system will serve to correct bad habits, reform the entire body and restore perfect health. (See Chapter VI.)

2. Proper Breathing

Without air man cannot live; it is his very life. A comprehensive understanding of the many uses of air in the body and the conscious direction of energy through the powers of the breath is a tremendous factor in the development of both physical and mental efficiency. Learn rhythmic breathing for health, power, poise, self-confidence and for a good digestion. (See Chapter III.)

3. Relaxation

The ability to relax at will and enjoy complete freedom from all physical strain and nervous tension is absolutely necessary for the maintenance of health and happiness and for the acquisition of mental power. It is the secret of perfect rest and restful sleep. The prevention of nervous or muscular tension increases all the natural powers and is most effective in the alignment of mind with brain power. Relaxation and flexibility are as essential to man as strength, and both add very materially to his endurance and nerve control. (See Chapter IV.)

4. Scientific Exercise

All depends upon *how* exercises or movements are performed. Unless properly executed they may easily do more harm than good. Speed, dexterity, and efficiency, together with muscle and nerve control, depend upon *flexibility* of the joints and muscles. The ligaments connecting the joints must be elastic and limber as well as strong, particularly those of the spinal vertebræ. It is necessary also that all joints be thoroughly and naturally lubricated. Long, elastic, flexible muscles far exceed short, knotty muscles in strength, quickness and endurance. They may be developed by proper exercise, work, posture, carriage, diet, breathing and by the use of will power, carefully directionalized. (See Chapters VI, VII, VIII and IX.)

5. Complete Elimination

All of the vital processes of the body include elimination, in one way or another. Thorough cleansing by natural elimination is one of the great secrets of health, whether through muscular exercise, the breath, the skin, the bowels, or the emotions or the mind. Elimination is a continuous function in the normal individual. The interference of any process of elimination is the dominant cause of disease and of nervous, mental and emotional disorders. The Indians resort to fasting, sun baths, sweat baths, mineral, mud, and hot and cold water baths, as an aid to elimination, along with certain herbs and foods of a loosening nature. An occasional internal water bath is helpful if properly taken. Regularity in habits of eating and of elimination is a law of health.

6. Proper Nourishment and Clothing

It is just as important to feed the human body scientifically as it is to take proper exercise. The body cells cannot build brain and brawn unless the blood is supplied with the proper materials with which to build them. It is equally impossible for nerves to function adequately when starved or when restricted in their operations by improper food or clothing. Keep the body fit by careful attention to diet. It is as necessary to health as education is to your brain development or your business.

7. Mental Control

Emotional and mental control by the power of will is man's greatest asset in the world today. The various effects of the emotions and passions are amazing in their scope. Man *is* what he *thinks;* he may become what he wills. Mental control of the body and the emotions spells power and success. Physical education with complete mental control along with an ethical influence is the ideal, all-around human development.

CHAPTER II

ABOUT INDIANS

Indian Prowess

Of all races in the world today the American Indian is the acknowledged superior in physical development. He possesses vigorous strength and yet is lithe, graceful and as straight as an arrow. He has the secret of keeping himself young, agile, strong and healthy, well into old age, and that without becoming senile. He can outrun the swiftest, outdistance the sturdiest, and always exhibits the most marvelous endurance.

What are his secrets of breathing? He never becomes exhausted or winded under the most trying circumstances.

How does he develop the long, lithe muscles, the sinuous strength, the freedom of every joint; is never muscle-bound, knotted or stiff? Though quiet, he is quick; his swift, certain movements display the strength and agility of a tiger.

How does he master himself so unflinchingly against the most cruel tortures? How does he gain the perfect control of facial expression, the control of tongue, temper, emotions, and mind? What secret underlies his perfectly controlled nerves and his stoical bravery?

He is balanced, poised and dignified, yet actively alert. How has he acquired such easy grace, such harmony of movement, such muscular control?

He is vibrant with vital power that emanates in subtle force from his calm and stoical exterior. His self-control is supreme. What powers are his for directionalizing the vital fluids and forces of his body? Of his mind? How does he develop that indomitable courage and fearlessness? How does he control his thoughts and will power? How does he master his mind?

The secret of his hidden powers lies in a certain knowledge of very definite laws—natural laws. All of these secrets and many more should be yours; they are the inherent right of every American.

The Indian has much to teach us. He is wise in the ways of Nature and has preserved a secret knowledge that is of great value to the white

7

man—knowledge without which he can never become thoroughly efficient or even truly civilized!

It is true that many Indians, forced to live as they are at the present time, in the narrow confines of Government Reservations, are not up to the standard of the Indian ideal, in fact have perceptibly deteriorated since their contact with the white man. Not all Indians are intellectual any more than are all people of any other race, but the more highly intelligent and spiritually-minded Indians possess a profound knowledge concerning the physical and mental powers of man. The pity of it is that the Indians are forgetting their own philosophy and rituals, and are being discouraged in their own valuable arts, especially their knowledge of herbs and Nature and the healing art in general.

Ages Old

For centuries the American Indian has practiced a system of body development which was handed down from the ages—antedating the Aztecs; legend has it before the Flood—from Atlantis. Recently unearthed bas-reliefs and statuary, hieroglyphs and rock paintings proclaim the red man's thorough knowledge of anatomical proportions, of scientific development and of carriage, as well as depicting feats of great skill and strength. Many of the famous Ju-jutsu tricks of the Japanese were known and practiced by Indians long before America was discovered. Their knowledge of the effects of sudden pressure upon certain nerve centers was preserved from antiquity.

Nature's Forces

The Indian is wise; having a great respect for Nature's powers and the elements, he investigates and learns how to apply them to his own use. For the same reason he carefully observes his "little brothers," the animals; he studies their marvelous instincts, powers, quickness, strength and endurance, then adapts their methods to his own needs.

He knows that it is foolish to waste energy, therefore he wisely conserves energy. He never makes a useless motion, each is studied, scientifically analyzed and necessary. He never goes through jerky, tensed exercises, they would not be useful to him. He never becomes "muscle-bound," as do our great athletes. He has a very *definite reason* for every move he makes. He saves himself all undue exertion—and this is often mistaken for laziness. He is economical and natural in the use of force and gets the greatest amount of power while expending the least amount of energy. His movements are quiet and rhythmic but efficient.

Child Training

From the time the tiny papoose is strapped on a board and carried upon his mother's back, his training begins. It is the business of the squaws to train the little ones and train them right. No carelessness is permitted, for each child is a ward of the entire tribe. He is taught self-control in infancy; to wait upon himself as soon as he is able; not to cry or whine when hurt or peeved; to control his facial expressions, and his feelings. He is trained to be fearless and courageous, morally clean and good humored, for it is the business of the tribe to rear "Braves" who can endure anything—and that without flinching—and, moreover, Braves who will make for health and happiness in their community.

As soon as the toddler is able to understand, he is taught to carry himself correctly; to walk, run, jump and dance, all according to definite rules. This becomes a habit long before he becomes a man.

The young Braves go through the most terrible and difficult endurance tests, for they must be stoical—mentally, emotionally and physically self-controlled—in order to be acknowledged as real men in the sight of their elders and their women.

Their manners, too are carefully cultivated according to tribal custom, for ceremonial law is strictly followed and it is requisite that they conduct themselves with becoming dignity and be a credit to their noble ancestors.

Indians are endowed with rare common sense. They encourage the use of games for both young and old, realizing their great value in making them strong, alert, mentally quick and active, and at the same time developing good humor and filling them with a joyous camaraderie. They are fully aware that in the hours of recreation come relaxation and the adjustment that counteracts later tension or mental strain. They consider the physical and mental development derived from sports, of far greater value than proficiency in the games themselves.

Indian Maidens

The young Indian girl is also put through a strenuous physical and mental training—for, otherwise, how could she teach her children or hope to rear Braves to be proud of? She is their constant and un-flinching example. Indian women do not neglect their children. The supple body of the young squaw makes child-bearing easy; she prepares for the ordeal (to her, a natural function) from childhood.

The Indian girl is an athlete and a sport. She is a daring rider, an expert swimmer, a crack shot and an adept with bow and arrow. She is also clever with her needle and mistress of basketry, bead work, pottery and the household arts. Moreover, she knows the secrets of successful farming and is capable of performing the hardest labor, quickly too, and with great ease and skill, displaying the most amazing endurance. Her soft, graceful curves conceal long, slender muscles of remarkable strength beneath the nut-brown smoothness of her natural, unspoiled skin.

The balancing power of the Zuni maiden is so perfect that she can carry a heavy water jug, poised upon her head, and *run* up the hundreds of rough-hewn steps to her lofty pueblo home, atop Acoma. Try carrying a water jug on your head for five miles! Her easy, steady gait with its sinuous roll at the hip-joint is very graceful.

With small, well-formed feet these light-footed children of the Sun step through the intricacies of a hundred graceful dances, in the most perfect harmony and rhythm—long, difficult dances, in which every movement of the head, eyes, hands and feet is studied and each motion of the supple body swings in harmony with every step while all are united to convey subtle interpretations filled with deep religious mean-ing. Not a sound of drum, not a note of lute or voice, nor the tiniest ornament worn by the dancers, but carries sacred significance. The squaws look with great disfavor upon American dancing and jazz, for to their minds it is not modest. Indian women are modest.

Ideals

They also have high ideals and aspirations. Their great teachers have taught them that sex is a sacred function and not to be degraded for mere emotional satisfaction. They are taught to recognize a great creative force or energy, and, aside from being a means for propagat-ing their race, a *power* to be transmuted into brain energy and used constructively for the benefit of their people.

The Indian Brave has observed that all animals are continent except in certain seasons, and he—he has a mind—he is greater than any animal—therefore he develops self-control. The Brave who has earned the right, may wear the long, pure feather of the white eagle at the crown of his head, an emblem of victory, of aspiration, of transmuted sex energy and of wisdom.[1]

Many secrets are his, which the white man does not yet understand and seldom believes but which, if he would study nature and her Laws, could understand and use to his great advantage.

The Indian's Philosophy of Life

The Indian's daily life is his religion. He *lives* what he thinks and believes. He is a *practical* psychologist. His philosophy of living is honest appreciation; he takes nothing for granted, and he is sincerely thankful for the common things of life.

His code is to be content with what he has and not want too much. He does not think he is entitled to Nature's gifts just because he wants them. Man's wants are legion—his needs are few.

He has no attachment to places or things.

He struggles toward perfection; he has one aim, one desire, one truth—and that is: TO LEARN.

When bathing, he blesses the stream and thanks the stream and God for water.

When picking a plant for food, he thanks it and is grateful while eating it, knowing it gives up its little life to sustain him.

When gathering herbs for medicine, he is reverent in that the herb sacrifices its life to save his.

For every move he makes, he knows that something suffers—so he never complains about suffering.

Among Indians the greatest respect is shown the aged. To them *it is obvious that with their years they must have gained wisdom out of experience.*

There is no such thing as prostitution in an Indian community. There is no double standard of morality. They have no poor houses and no orphan asylums. Orphans are adopted by friends of the parents and immediately assume an equal right with the children of the new household.

[1] "That the Quiches possessed the key to regeneration is evident from an analysis of the symbols appearing upon the images of their Priests and Gods." Symbolical Philosophy, by Manly P. Hall.

Indian marriages are usually successful and the couple grow old in harmony with each other and their children.

An important feature of the red man's psychology is that he never acts hastily or through impulse, but only after deep thought and consideration, weighing all sides of a problem. The Indian is not easily fooled. His discrimination is highly developed, for he is fully aware that he must seek guidance from his higher consciousness *within himself*. He is therefore not easily influenced by outward appearances.

He accepts responsibility with full labor and adversity with great patience; he argues that he must have deserved them or they would not be his.

He masters pain and emotion with self-control, and courageously meets his problems in life. And his problem is greater now than it has ever been.

He well knows that it is not enough merely to believe; he must *act*.

He incorporates natural, ethical and physical law into his very being, he makes them part of his daily life, the basis of his religion, and the foundation of his home. This is the essence of his whole psychology and his philosophy of living, and the very core of his being. It is true Brotherhood.

> *He serves Life through his body.*
> *He serves Nature through his mind.*
> *He serves God through his will.*

The Indian's psychology of life is peace and it was only when he felt the lash, the bullet and the sword of the white man that he stood at bay and fought for his rights and his freedom—in his own native land. The very thing that we "intruders" sought for ourselves in his beautiful and free America we have denied the first American! The Indian was forced to become an alien in the land in which he was born!

And now for many years the Indians of America, dozens of tribes, whether Mohawk, Seminole, Iroquois or Zuni, have, alike, all buried their hatchets. They live in peace and in silence. The white man could follow the red man's example with considerable profit. The Indian is not a savage; he has laid aside his tomahawk, he no longer seeks the scalp-locks of his erstwhile selfish enemy—the white man.

Would that the white man could learn to forget the hideous might of his horrible warfare of guns, gas, shells and commercialism, beside which Indian warfare was tame and puerile, and smoke a National Pipe of Peace with the Indian and an International Pipe of Peace with the world!

CHAPTER III

THE POWERS OF THE BREATH

The fact that the breath is of greater importance than food is fully recognized by the Indians. Not only is breathing the most important function of the body, but all other functions are dependent upon it. Man can subsist many days without food, but he can live only a few minutes without air. Respiration is a function of the body that is continuous and without cessation. The purification of the blood by air in the lungs and the propelling of that blood by the heart to the farthest extremities of the body, and back again, depend upon the breath. When respiration ceases, all the vital functions cease and death ensues.

Since the lungs are situated in the torso above the diaphragm, protected by a bony cage composed of the ribs, shoulders, spine and breast bones, and not in the abdomen, the Indian claims that the breath should *not* be drawn toward the abdominal region. The muscles of the diaphragm are designed to operate *up* and *down,* rather than in and out. This action is in harmony with an inward and upward pull of the abdominal muscles. Properly used, the diaphragm is capable of infinitely more power. It certainly sounds reasonable and furthermore it works. In our humble opinion, many large abdomens are due to abdominal breathing and rigid postures. The spine, ribs, shoulders and breast bones are all designed for flexible movement, to coordinate with the rhythmic motion of the breath. Nature abhors rigidity.

Man also breathes through the pores of the skin and through the tiny spaces between the cells. The human body is porous.

Oxygen starvation, from the lack of pure air and sunshine, or from insufficient breathing, is more common by far than food starvation. It is starvation in the midst of plenty, through carelessness or ignorance.

The white man should breathe more and eat less. The average person uses only one-sixth of his lung capacity; he only half lives!

Food cannot be digested or assimilated without the action of air in the process. Deep breathing assists very materially in producing both health and strength. It serves to increase the weight of thin, emaciated persons or those wasted with disease, and also aids in the reduction of excessive fat, through proper oxygenation.

Fresh Air

Breathing stale or devitalized air is suicidal; it contains quantities of poisonous gases and is absolutely lacking in electrical energy. Fresh air contains an abundance of sun or life force without which nothing can exist. The living cells of the body obtain their electric life essence through the air from the sun. It is small wonder that the Indians worship the Power of the Sun, the source of their very life, the manifested symbol of their Sun God, the Power behind the Sun, "The One about whom nothing may be said." When the white man teaches his child, as the Indian does, that the air he breathes, the water he drinks, the food he eats and the thoughts he thinks are all charged with sparks of vital energy, and that in order to absorb that life-force into his body he must live in harmony with Nature, using her boundless resources in their primitive freshness, then and only then will the white race become as sturdy as the red race.

The air contains those vital constituents or units of energy, electric life sparks, residing in the heart of every atom. It is life-force itself— derived from the life-principle of the sun. Whether deprived consciously or unconsciously of this principle, force or energy, the rhythms are disturbed and the health and vitality of any living creature suffers thereby.

There are two breath rhythms, major and minor; in addition we have rhythms in the heart pulsations which are dependent upon the breath. Breathing in and out, when understood, can keep the body in a state of health and harmony and the mind in a state of controlled equilibrium. Breathing constitutes a double rhythm. It is exercised not only by the lungs but by the skin in a constant inpouring and outpouring of subtle hidden forces carried through the air. Radio has made us realize much.

Man resembles the radio except that he is a broadcasting station as well as a receiving station, a transmitter and loud speaker all in one. He is capable of sending and receiving both radio-electric and telepathic messages. Unfortunately his mental crystal occasionally develops flaws and he frequently becomes static—just like any other radio!

Interesting Facts

The Indian knows many interesting facts about the breath and breathing; among them the following are highly interesting to us.

Life enters the body with the incoming breath and departs with the outgoing breath. This is true of man, animals and plants.

The breath is automatically controlled by the mind, through certain sense centers in the brain.

The breath is suspended in lifting, pulling, pushing, or pressing.

The breath is first inhaled, then held, then exhaled when excreting or expelling anything from the body.

Electricity, the life agent or carrier, together with oxygen, is attracted into the blood by iron, and serves to sustain and promote cell growth, while the electric *force* itself is used in the emotions, thoughts and will power. This produces growth. But if the blood is deficient in iron it naturally cannot attract enough oxygen for its purification.

The blood uses oxygen from the air while the nervous system uses a certain electrical force radiated by the sun and contained in the ethers —called by the East Indians, Prana. The life-giving force expands while the physical or natural force contracts into form. This is true of body cells as well as thought-forms.

Man alternates in polarity with every breath. He accumulates force, or he relaxes, often unconsciously and imperceptibly, with the influx or efflux of his breath. He may adjust his polarity to breathing and thereby control the life current, making it positive or negative at will. When properly understood, this process may be used for self-healing. It is a matter of will power, together with the understanding of very definite laws. It is quite contrary to self-hypnotism. There is a great difference between the states of negative passivity and positive receptivity. It is dangerous to make oneself receptive to unknown powers without full knowledge of their operations.

One nostril is used for the positive and the other for the negative life currents. Many Indians understand this process thoroughly. Indian adepts and healers are intimately acquainted with many mysterious and powerful rhythms of the body and manipulate and control them by the power of will through mind.

It is through breathing, in and out, and through the heart pulsations that both food and water are utilized in the body. With such interferences as tight clothing, belts, hat bands, cramped positions, bad habits of posture or carriage, the actions of rhythmic breathing and fluid circulation and rhythm are disturbed or checked and the vitality of the body is lowered. Lack of sunshine and air, insufficient or improper methods of exercise, unbalanced diet and uncontrolled thoughts gnaw at the root of a healthful civilization.

Man is naturally flooded by the constant vibratory rate of the world, with each breath, and with the special vibratory rates of his particular environment. The Indian endeavors to make or control his own environment. To accomplish this he combines thought with effort.

The powers of the breath relative to speech, creation and "the word made flesh" have a highly significant meaning among the Indians. They know the laws of voice placement, and control their vocal chords with amazing skill. A whoop or yell can be made to carry miles or echo and reëcho a number of times. That he uses healing mantrams is well known.

Ordinary man cannot permanently stop the action of breathing by will but *he can control its effects upon his body, emotions and mind.*

Skin Breathing

One of the most important offices of the skin is breathing. The outer coat of skin has millions upon millions of tiny valve-like openings called pores, each provided with minute muscles which serve to open and close them. The skin is so porous as to be penetrable by light, heat, color, sound and moisture. Air enters the pores carrying the electric life-giving currents into the body, where it is immediately taken up by the blood. Radio-electric messages also reach the nerves through the pores of the skin.

Perspiration

There are two kinds of perspiration or sweat, visible and invisible. The visible perspiration carries poisons, excretions and refuse out through the pores of the skin in the form of moisture. The invisible perspiration, noticeable in body odors, exudes in the form of poisonous gases or fumes. It is easy therefore to understand how important it is to perspire. The natural perspiration produced by exercise should not be checked in any way, for muscular exertion throws off poisons and is extremely beneficial. With a moderate amount of cleanliness there should be no offensive odors, provided that intestinal elimination is normal and the diet correct.

If the pores become clogged with dirt, grease, powder or any sort of exuded waste matter, or if the muscular action of the pores is weakened so that they cannot open and close quickly and easily, they become sluggish and unable to perform their exceedingly important functions. Under such circumstances reabsorption of the poisons and gases is the result with serious injury to the blood stream and the nerves.

If the blood stream is affected, every organ and nerve in the body is deprived of pure air and adequate nourishment—with self-poisoning as the inevitable result. This is especially true when the vital organs, particularly the lungs, heart, liver, kidneys, brain and sex organs, are overworked and weakened. In order to have a healthy body and an active skin it is absolutely necessary to have pure, clean blood. This necessitates clean digestive organs and intestines—particularly a clean colon. If you will keep these members clean, Nature will take care of the skin, provided you keep the surface clean and eat and think properly. The nerves beneath the outer skin are superlatively sensitive and send their messages with acute irritability when improperly nourished. Many nervous cases may be traced to insufficient breathing either through the lungs or the skin.

Yogi Breathing

Fancy, skip-stop, "occult" methods of breathing, with concentration on the solar plexus or other nerve centers are not advisable; in fact, they may prove very dangerous to the white race.

There is a mysterious "inner breath" known to a few highly developed American Indians and practiced by them when going through fire, under water, through dense smoke or during profound spiritual meditation. With this method they do not employ the lungs but directionalize the life force through the spinal nerve centers to the brain, using the pneumogastric nerve! Yogis or Indian seers, who understand their nervous anatomy, often obtain remarkable results, but white peoples, who are not thoroughly familiar with cell life and growth, or with the vital nerve centers and the various forces that flow through the body—many of which operate with tremendous hidden power— *should not play with fire.* The insane asylums contain many who *thought they knew* or who have experimented out of curiosity. Natural growth through a process of normal development while living a pure life is the only safe or sane method.

Air Hygiene

Any kind of building, office, or dwelling, should be given a thorough air bath several times a day, to make it fit to live in.

It is much easier to heat rooms filled with fresh air than with stale air.

Window curtains, drapes and portières should have rings sewed to them so that they may be slid back or fastened away from the windows and doors when airing the rooms. Window shades should not be drawn over the open windows in the sleeping room.

Bed drapes are not healthful, they catch dust and germs.

Open the windows wide at night and have plenty of fresh air circulating through your bedroom. Do not be afraid of night air! It is the only air there is to breathe at night.

Open gas heaters are dangerous unless provided with an outlet pipe to carry away the burned fumes. Burned gas fumes are poisonous and deadly.

A room in which any sort of heater that consumes oxygen is burning—even an oil reading lamp—should have a circulation of fresh air constantly coming in and through it, otherwise the oxygen and vital electric forces of the air are soon consumed and the air becomes devitalized and vitiated.

The exhaled breath, consisting of carbon dioxide and other poisonous exhalations, laden with disease germs, of several persons in a poorly ventilated room, is decidedly dangerous to health.

It is well known that the nostrils are designed to filter, purify and warm the air, and have fine hairs growing inside to protect the delicate membranes and to prevent dirt, insects and destroyer-germs from entering the passages and lungs. Mouth-breathing attracts disease, causes throat troubles, catarrh, susceptibility to colds and many other infections, together with inflammation of the respiratory tract. It is a disgusting habit and should be corrected immediately. Children should be taught to breathe through the nostrils. Tilt the head slightly forward, when sleeping, to keep the lips closed, and lie on the side. Tobacco smoke pollutes the air and is injurious to lung tissue. It is injurious to the teeth and causes a bad breath; it wrecks the nerves eventually. Never sleep in a room where anyone has been smoking without first airing it thoroughly.

Always admit sunshine, through open windows when possible. It is filled with electrical life force and purifies the air. Dark rooms and houses are not healthful and soon become musty and dank.

Sleeping porches are excellent. It would be well if everyone could sleep out of doors.

How Indians Breathe

Proper breathing during the performance of all exercises is of the greatest importance. Do not attempt strenuous movement while inhaling. Inhale first and then make the move. It is advisable to take a full breath once or twice between exercises.

The Full Breath

EXERCISE 1.—This exercise develops the lungs and increases their capacity; it promotes diaphragmatic control and develops the chest. Using the entire lung capacity, as given in the full breath, it is both healthful and stimulating. A regular, rhythmic breath, taking the same number of moments to inhale, to hold, and to exhale, without jerking or forcing the breath or the respiratory organs, is the normal way to breathe.

Upon rising in the morning stand before an open window and inhale deeply ten full breaths, in the following manner:

Inhale.—Keep the mouth closed. Begin at the diaphragm a little below the waist-line, and gradually draw the air up into the lungs at the lower ribs, expanding toward the sides; then up into the chest and still higher up toward the shoulders and collar-bones, filling the upper lobes of the lungs, counting 10. As the air fills the upper portion of the lungs, the diaphragm will lift naturally and the muscles of the abdomen will draw inward and up. Hold and count 10. The same number of seconds should elapse between breaths as when inhaling or exhaling.

Exhale.—Still holding the chest firmly, allow the pressure while exhaling to come first from the abdomen, drawing the muscles slightly in and up, then gradually expel the air—all of it. Count 10. Relax the chest and abdomen.

The diaphragm will act automatically to inhale the next breath.

Practice this full breath many times daily, whenever you think of it, and soon you will have established the habit of correct breathing and the body will be immensely toned thereby. Full rhythmic breathing of pure, fresh, cold air is enormously refreshing; it stimulates both body and mind to action. When practiced in the open air and sunshine it acts like a tonic. When mildly practiced, with the thoughts and emotions subdued, it has a calming and restful influence.

When employed in ordinary work, the breath need not be inhaled to the entire lung capacity but it should be complete, always using the diaphragm and the upper and lower lungs. This method gently massages the vital organs and strengthens them by moving them in rhythmic harmony, and greatly assists digestion and assimilation.

If a feeling of dizziness is experienced when first practicing the full breath, be assured that it is much needed, for it is an indication of weakness, through disuse, of the lungs and the muscles which support them. Practice frequently, and by degrees increase the lung capacity.

If you have been in the habit of breathing in the old way, with the diaphragm moving in and out instead of up and down, it would help to place your hands on the abdomen and test the action.

Indians breathe deeply and rhythmically and therefore require much less food than the white man. They think constructively and send life-force throughout the body by will with the breath.

Clean the Lungs

EXERCISE 2.—Fill the lungs to capacity, using the full breath, then blow three times, on the one breath, expelling the air with force. Exhale thoroughly to be sure that the lungs are entirely empty. The muscles of the abdomen and diaphragm will draw inward and up suddenly and powerfully with each blow. This breath is very invigorating and, if used when fatigued, will increase the circulation and produce a warm glow over the entire body. At the same time it cleanses every crevice of the lungs, dispelling all stale air, and develops the muscles.

Overdevelopment of the lungs often enlarges and strains them, and is also dangerous because of enforced heart action. Do not strain overhard with any exercise and remember always that a slow, steady, even development alone is desirable.

CHAPTER IV

MENTAL CONTROL

We live in the world we think in.
We make environment by thought.
We make character by thought.
We destroy with wrong thoughts.
We build with constructive thoughts.

Is it not a glorious satisfaction that, no matter where we are, or under what conditions we labor, we can think as we please? No matter what our state of consciousness or environment, no matter what our exterior conditions, no matter what the thoughts of others may be or what they do to influence us, *we have always the power to think what we will!* Thoughts are free. We choose any kind we wish. Thoughts have the power to calm the storms of mind instantly—or to ruffle its peace. The great thing is to exclude the undesirable thoughts, to give them no place. Reason is the governor of the machine. We have faculties, but do not use them; we have the equipment, but remain unaware. Of our forty odd faculties less than eight are used by the majority; we run along on less than eight-fortieths of our mental power most of the time and skid terribly. With the generation of a little more will power we could sit in the driver's seat and control.

Every emotion has the impress of mind behind it, consciously or unconsciously, either from our own minds or from others. Every movement of muscle or nerve, whether voluntary or involuntary, is directed by a subtle influence or a suggestion of mind. If you will study yourself carefully, you will observe that every motion and move-ment; every feeling, worthy or unworthy; every emotion, good or bad; every glow of health and every blight of disease has its origin in some kind of *desire*. Desire holds sway over the mind. But WILL governs the mental processes and is capable of guiding the desires. Learn to guard the kind and quality of your desires and you will know the Indian's secret of mental self-control.

The greatest benefits are received only when mind and body work together in harmony and coördination, with the mind directing the body and the desires guiding the will. Muscles are organs of will. Man effects all his material accomplishments through muscular control. If the muscles are underdeveloped or allowed to become weak and flabby, that interval between good intentions and their accomplishment widens insurmountably. Every change of thought and feeling plays upon the muscles in subtle ways.

The world today regards ease and lounging, with nothing to do, as desirable. The Indians, along with the ancient Greeks, believed it a most dangerous state. Plato advised his students to "Make good use of every idle moment." If idle moments were given over to constructive thought, great things could be accomplished, for, if we think about a thing earnestly enough and long enough, we are bound to produce certain results—good or evil.

We are forced into artificial exercise because we are not living naturally; we do not use our bodies as we should. We have practically given up all sorts of manual labor. We only exercise the body, for the most part, because we have to in order to be well. Sometimes we even begrudge that time, fearing that we will not be making money—fearing also that we may have to keep up the bothersome exertion else grow sick or fat. Of course this is due to a false mode of living. We do not develop naturally, like the Indian. All falseness is forced to pay a price; that is the penalty the body pays.

But the mind also pays a price and it is a heavy one. The failures and ills of the body act upon the mind and deteriorate its efficiency. The mind again reacts upon the body, and so, back and forth, until the poor human creature is a nervous or physical wreck with a mind that can no longer function with any degree of accuracy. It is impossible for the mind to function dependably through taut or irritated nerves. Nerves cannot register accurately when excited or sick; sensations are not carried to the brain correctly nor is mental instruction directed to various parts of the body normally, and the subject is rendered abnormal or subnormal. In this condition FEAR descends with terrible force upon the individual. He loses control over his own thoughts and his will power vanishes.

It is right here that the Indian's rule of life is so strong. It is so simple that any child can learn it. He is taught how to control any thought of fear from infancy. By the time he is a youth he has no fear, does not know the use or meaning of cowardly fear. He has learned to balance extremes with a certain rhythm of thought. He knows the art of thought-rhythm and its effects upon his body and all its functions, upon his emotions and feelings, and their subsequent reactions upon the body and the mind.

The Indian's secret of self-control lies in this; while he does not show impatience, anger or fear, he does something infinitely more— he does not even permit himself to *feel* these emotions. By the power of will, with a quick control of thought, he changes any evil or negative thought-force (for thought is a force) into a good, positive thought-force. He compels his mind to obey his will. He thinks what he *wills*—not what he *feels*. Thus he actually changes his feelings in the process. He compels his mind, by the power of his will, to think brave, good or positive thoughts and the *power* of such thoughts actually transforms his feelings. It is a simple but a potent alchemy. In this way the lower passions and emotions are transmuted into the highest aspirations. In the same way emotion may be changed into purpose, feeling may be made over into a constructive power, and the fiery fevers of unrest and irritable nervousness may be made to become a propelling force, while the madness of hate or anger may be transformed into the supreme poise and balance of perfect tolerance.

Stop, when filled with passionate emotion. Be Still. Listen! Listen to the higher aspirations within yourself and give them a chance to guide you sensibly and normally. Anger and hate are not normal— they are sub-normal—animal. It is only when normal poise has been sufficiently recovered that the mind is capable of thinking or reasoning, and not until then. The subject or cause of the emotional upheaval may, by that time, be approached from an entirely different angle.

Compel the mind, by the power of will, to think good, patient, calm thoughts, through reasoning. *Know* that the *power* is within you, supplied from an infinite source. Know that the only limitation is the limiting idea or thought about it! *Will power is free.* Everyone is at liberty to help himself. You may draw upon it to the uttermost capacity of your being. You need it when filled with fear-thoughts or anger-thoughts, for they react like subtle poisons upon the body. Realize this; there is no such thing as fear or anger. It is only a thought in mind, a personal attitude. Change the thought or mental attitude, and the thing called fear vanishes!

Cast out destructive thoughts the moment they enter your mind. Give them no place, nor allow them a moment's foothold. Fill the mind, at once, with the opposite kind of thoughts. One or the other will dominate and rule. Both cannot occupy the mind at the same time. It is entirely up to the thinker *which* will dominate. Learn to concentrate on the desired thought to the exclusion of all other thoughts or feelings. Make a mental picture of the condition desired, idealize it and then work to hold it. The will is no less dependent upon the culture it receives than is the body or the mind. Learn to cultivate and control the will.

Consistent thinking will build a consistent mind and produce adequate works with lasting effects upon the thinker. Learn to correlate works with knowledge, thoughts with feelings, acts with desires. Think, compare and study their correspondences. Ideals are essential, but something more is required; a carrying through into action and making practical in the daily life.

From early childhood the Indian is taught to recognize the lesson in everything, in every contact and experience. The meaning of each circumstance to himself, however small. This is of first importance. Even young children are taught to consider, reflect, meditate and apply the moral lesson to themselves. They are taught not to act thoughtlessly; not to give way to impulse; not to express every chance thought or notion that enters their minds. They are taught the value of silence and to think things out to a conclusion quietly without voicing random opinions. And this is not accomplished by repression. Repression is negative and carries a fear-thought with its recoil. It is like a spring, pressed down and held for a time, but which leaps forth with accumulated power when released, controlling the repressor. All fears, passions and slavish habits must be *overcome*—not repressed. A complete change of attitude and thought, held to vigorously and tenaciously, will overcome all adverse conditions, and every difficulty will succumb to your inner power. In this way *obstacles become a means to growth; hindrances become opportunities* for gaining strength of character and self-control. When an obstacle presents itself, instead of allowing a fear-thought to stay in the mind, change your attitude at once and look upon the seeming obstacle as an opportunity, and work around it and over it and under it, and thereby gain just so much additional strength in its management!

Anyone may follow the Indian's ancient wisdom and bring about harmony, peace, success and satisfactory progress in his outer life, if he desires fervently to improve himself; to improve his inner life and thought and discipline his mind. "As a man thinketh, so is he." The wise man idealizes and aspires ardently within and becomes outwardly what he wills.

No matter what activity the Indian undertakes, he follows certain rules of thought. The process of thinking correlates directly with the action. A flash of thought accompanies each move. This method should be used when directionalizing the action of the muscles in the exercises given in this book. Remember: *energy follows thought*.

Indian Methods

1. The Indian breathes deeply and rhythmically, maintaining a faith and confidence in a limitless supply of power; his to use *constructively*.

2. He uses the muscles of his body and applies his certain knowledge of an inner spiritual strength, which strength or power is immediately imparted to the muscles. He *knows* this power is within him.

3. He *thinks* with each act. He *wills* with each thought. Every action carries a constructive thought behind it; thus, will and power accompany every motion. In this way a directionalized thought-force, vibrant with life-force, actually enters the cells of the body, giving them a power and potency ordinarily undreamed of.

4. He concentrates his mind on Infinite Good, and floods his being with a desire to be, to do, to become something greater than he is. He works for what he gets, mentally and physically; he does not expect something for nothing.

5. He makes his mind one with the laws of Nature—obediently subservient—and *compels* his emotions and his body to follow these laws. He does not expect God or Nature to change the law to suit his whims or his needs.

6. He practices concentration, too, and brings his mind by power of will to one-pointedness. He will not permit his thoughts to flit about like a flea; he holds them steady, brings them back with forceful will power to the subject he wishes to think about and holds them steady. He ponders and considers a question from every angle. He is never in uncertain haste; he must be sure before he will act, sure that he is right and with the law. Otherwise he knows well he is foredoomed to failure—eventually.

7. He practices meditation. He seeks a quiet place and enters upon a fast. He makes peace with his God and the divine part of himself,

confesses his own shortcomings to himself and endeavors to question himself as to his motives and his thoughts, desires and actions. These he goes over carefully in his mind for hours—sometimes days. Then he meditates upon the great principles of Good, Love, Truth, Honor, and the Laws of the Universe as expressed in Nature and himself. He tries to know or understand his God through learning about or understanding himself and his fellow men.

Agility, strength and superhuman endurance are the rewards of his body.

Power, poise and self-conquest are the fruits of his mental control.

Confidence, faith and an inner peace are the expression of his spirit.

Mental Gymnastics for the Earnest Student

Get over the idea of hurry, hustle and excitement.

Practice being calm, cool, quiet and poised.

Stop to think before talking or answering. Ask yourself: Is it true? Is it kind? Is it necessary?

Do not wear yourself out with useless chatter or talk for hours about nothing in particular. You cannot afford to waste time or energy. Apply that precious force to self-improvement or to doing some good.

Be constructive; be creative; get ahead; get somewhere with yourself—*within*.

Do not worry about what has not happened—and probably never will.

Do not worry about what *may* happen. In fact do not worry at all. It is the most wearing, exhausting, ageing, useless pastime invented to torture the mind and soul of man. Rather, make a mental picture of the ideal, imagining the thing or condition that would be best for all concerned.

Cultivate a creative, ideal mentality. We must have something to look forward to—dreams of future greatness or achievement of some sort. Riches and material things do not satisfy. When attained they do not make us happy. We need ideals—ideals more powerful than we are. We must *be* something within in order to be truly happy. Formulate ideals of what you wish to do; of what you wish to become.

Make the most of your natural opportunities. "Seek and ye shall find" them.

Concentrate your mind upon a subject and use strong determination to bring the mind back forcefully every time the thoughts wander.

Learn to guide the thoughts along any desired channel by using will power.

Study your motive for action, making sure that it is good, else it will turn upon you like a boomerang when you are unaware.

Sit quietly, and force yourself to think, weigh and consider your own problems, looking at them mentally from all angles.

Study the possible effects of the proposed action.

Study the effects of your action upon others.

Study out what you could do in event of failure.

Cultivate a positive state of mind while directing the thoughts in the line desired, but keep the convictions open and fluidic, allowing for possible changes of opinion as the thought process evolves and grows into form.

Bodily restlessness is one of the great faults of the present generation. This conquered, mental restlessness, along with irregular impulses will be half conquered, too.

Do not permit yourself to become discouraged. Feel certain of success. Maintain a determined, steadfast, unalterable resolution and you cannot fail to develop your mental powers, your soul, and your body.

CHAPTER V

THE ART OF RELAXATION

"Walk in the rhythm of life;
Your limbs will not tire.
Sing with the rhythm of life;
Your voice will gain sweetness.
Dance in the rhythm of life;
Your feet will not touch the ground.
Breathe in rhythm.
Think in rhythm.
Talk in rhythm.
Sing in rhythm.
Dance in rhythm.
Let rhythmic be your life."
East Indian.*

Perfect relaxation is an art and one which everyone should know and be able to practice at will, both *physically and mentally*. Mind and body both require periods of rest or recreation as much as they need sleep. Frequently a change of occupation will rest the body; a change of thought will rest the mind. Relaxation, like rest and repose, builds up the pliability leading to stamina and alertness.

Action and Reaction Are Equal

All creatures require a period of rest for readjustment following a period of activity; one follows the other as day follows night. Man obeys the law of rhythmic periodicity of alternate action and reaction quite naturally, but without giving it much thought. The Indians of antiquity were not so matter-of-course—they sought to understand the values of such an exact law and its application to themselves. They recognized the fact that the body does not blindly run itself but is subject to certain laws and forces which act in harmony with each other. They realized also that physical and mental harmony are possible only when the conditions are right and life is conducted in accordance with

* Paramananda.

29

Nature and immutable law. So, with them, relaxation and rest came to have as much significance as their activities. Hence the Indian system of physical education allows for those necessary periods of relaxation both in the exercises themselves and in the parts of the body employed during the various movements. It provides for rhythmic periods of action and relaxation and for the systematic use of certain muscles with the relaxation of certain other muscles at the same time. This makes both work and exercise much easier for their accomplishment is without strain or unnecessary tensing. It teaches the great art of relaxing at will.

Make Life Easier

All work and no play is devitalizing. All play and no work is demoralizing. A happy combination of the two is essential to normal living. Constant "driving" of oneself or "going on one's nerves" will inevitably result in shattered nerves, disease, or mental deficiency. "For every period of intense effort the mind must be compensated by a similar period of relaxation." * A life of pleasure-seeking inhibits the growth of character, it stunts the growth of mind. Some people work harder seeking pleasure and amusement than the day-laborer in a ditch. The penalty is more severe than from overwork. It spells spiritual death. Mind and will must be used in order to truly live.

Nervous Tension

While one of the commonest of human ailments, nervous tension is not only one of the most baffling to cope with, but one of the most difficult to overcome. Its effects upon the body and mind are almost endless in variety and scope, being the primary cause of many disorders, whether directly or indirectly. Strain on the muscles and nerves is one of the great destroyers.

Nervous tension is capable of disorganizing the entire digestive system to an alarming degree and frequently inhibits both assimilation and elimination. It affects the brain, the spine and the various nerve plexes. Repressed or restricted forces are bottled up only to explode later in some sort of emotional outburst, sex debauch, disease, or, worse still, mental unbalance.

Nervous tension immediately tightens every muscle and nerve in

* Lectures on Ancient Philosophy: An Introduction to the Study and Application of Rational Procedure. Manly P. Hall.

the body and restricts the normal action and free and rhythmic flow of the various circulations. It holds the poisons in the body preventing their free exudation and by their presence creates more poisons. It prevents the free flow of any kind of force or energy to or from the body. It prohibits by constriction the circulation of fluids, ethers, air or gases through the tiny conduits so delicately and marvelously constructed to convey these forceful elements.

Further, with nervous tension, anxiety, or fear, we unconsciously build up a strong resistance to the entrance of those finer forces of nature, the strengthening and purifying ethers of the atmosphere, the impulsion of life-force itself, and cut ourselves off from the very source of endless supply, the natural reservoir of universal life and energy. When we permit ourselves to get into a state of tense nervousness or nervous tension we are only half alive! The nerves hold fast, resist, and cannot report correctly because they are in a state that makes them incapable of adjustment to vibratory rates. Everything becomes distorted, colored with fear, anxiety or apprehension, and the resultant impressions are not reliable. The nerves can neither receive nor send nervo-grams easily or dependably and are in no sense true indicators of facts. This condition also upsets emotional impressions, both coming and going, for nerve-force is both introactive and reactive. Hence, when tensed in body we become tensed in mind. When the brain is subjected to nervous tension either through action or reaction, we can neither think, reason, nor remember; for the mind cannot function adequately through a disordered vehicle.

Causes

Now let us see if we can get at the causes of this bugbear of modern civilization. What are they? An intense, strained, holding fast to—what? Various notions, mental irritants, worries, fears and what not! And for what purpose, and to what end? When we stop long enough to face the situation honestly we are forced to realize that it is all in the mind—nothing but a distorted mental attitude. It is all foolishness, too, and *very* aging. Learn to relax mentally in order to relax physically.

Fear and Worry

Little children seldom know the meaning of fear until taught by their elders. Their faith and confidence in a higher protective power is not questioned for a moment. They are taught fear with every natural impulse to investigate their surroundings—fear of a bogie man, the dark, injury, people, and an endless array of what must seem to them—horrors. It grows all too easily into a habit and finally seems a reality. Fear and worry are like a terrible disease when they fasten their tentacles into the heart and mind. They inhibit the power to think! They paralyze the ability to analyze or reason. They are the greatest hindrance to relaxation and rest in the world. *Worry* is an exaggerated imagination concerning the things or conditions one fears. It displays a lack of confidence in the ability of the Supreme Power to manipulate correctly the laws of the universe, laws conceived, executed and guided by Him. Fear is purely a mental concept, the fabrication of a diseased imagination that gives more power to evil than to good. If that were possible all would be chaotic—nothing but disorder and confusion. Either there is a Great and Munificent Power of All Good—or there isn't! If there is not, then all should be chaos—without law or order! But this is not the case. Law and order abound in the whole magnificent universe of suns, moons, stars and our little earth. A gorgeous round of days, nights, seasons, and a multiplicity of powerful forces demonstrate the truth of Absolute Law, every moment of life. Once you get this great and satisfactory truth thoroughly in mind and *know* it way down in the depths of your being, a sense of peace and trust will be yours, giving wing to fear and worry. To attain any degree of happiness requires that we rely upon That, the One All-Power, Good—by whatever name you wish to call it, it is the same. Rely upon It implicitly and with unbending faith. Each must reason this out for himself and arrive at his own conclusion within his own mind before he can know the true meaning of happiness.

The greatest secret of relaxation is simply to overcome fear and worry and self-pity thoughts—in the mind. It is then, and then only, that we can let go. Being destructive, they are disintegrating in their effects. They steal hours of precious time from much worthier pursuits. We have no time to waste, for, in order to be successful, keep young and be happy we must give all our energy to constructive thoughts; keep high in faith; and allow reason, intuition, and conscience a chance to operate more efficiently.

There are several ways to go about overcoming the fear-worry habit. Following are a few suggestions that have proved successful in difficult cases.

Music

The power of soft melodious music is wonderfully soothing to jaded nerves and tensed bodies. It has been repeatedly demonstrated that harmonious rhythmic tones so affect the vibratory rates of nerve force as to subdue raging, wild animals, quiet the violently insane, heal nervous disorders and cure the sick. We believe that there is a great future in both harmony and color for curative purposes. The opposite in music is also quite true; discordant sounds irritate, sensuous music excites, certain rhythms produce lethargy. Certain sounds or rates of vibration, constantly repeated, have been known to produce insanity. A weak mind has not sufficient power to counteract the effect or rise above it.

To go through a number of graceful, rhythmic movements, keeping time to beautiful, cheerful music is a great help in regaining self-control. With children or invalids this is the quickest and easiest way.

Dancing is also a means to nervous relaxation and a relief from mental strain—especially interpretive dancing, using the imagination, idealizing joy and happiness. (See Dancing, Chapter XI.)

Laughter

"Laughter is good for the soul." It must be for it makes for happiness. We grown-ups are too apt to go through life seriously. We forget how to laugh. We forget the joyous freedom of childhood with its happy laughter and spontaneous humor. We forget even to smile and too often frighten those who approach us with our grim sternness. Too often we snicker or sneer when we do give vent to some sort of humor and indulge in the laughter of sophistication—a humor that requires the discomfort of another for its fullest enjoyment. Too bad. We forget to be kind. Laughter at another's expense must react upon ourselves eventually, for it sets up a sort of poison in the system with its cruel thoughtlessness of another's suffering.

Wholesome, joyous laughter is purifying and cleansing in its effects—it purges both mind and body of its dull vibrations. Everyone feels better after a good laugh. If you would relax—learn to laugh. Laugh heartily and good-humoredly. If we "could see ourselves as others see us" the laugh would be on us. Try it. Try to see yourself as you are, with all your funny little habits and ways, funny ideas about things you know nothing about, and see yourself, for a change, as a ridiculous clown in cap and bells, making a fool of yourself before the world—and not knowing it! See the funny side of it and you cannot help laughing. It is "good for the soul" to see ourselves thus—and laugh off our own seriousness about ourselves. As a people, we need to develop a better sense of humor along with much better manners, more tolerance, a gracious demeanor and more kindness of speech. In trying to be funny we cut deep, regardless of the other fellow's feelings.

The Business of Life

We try to run life like a business, these days, and in so doing we are merely succeeding in taking all of the joy out of it. We lose all spontaneity as we grow up and scarcely dare to be natural. Our muscles along with our nerves become atrophied, until we cannot relax. We take ourselves too seriously. We are so anxious to become important in the world; more anxious to impress others with our importance. We become obsessed with our own concepts and make life hard for ourselves. We imagine ourselves very necessary in the scheme of things. We forget that one day the flags of a nation are at half-mast and the next day finds a readjustment with slight variation in formula—and things go on just the same!

That "I am holier than thou" attitude is a dangerous state of mind. It develops conceit. It would be well to consider that no matter how far we advance, the path of improvement stretches endlessly ahead. Self-satisfaction is the insurmountable obstacle in the path of true progress.

People who worry, fuss, and fume make life miserable for everyone about them. They worry others and make them worry, too, when they might have been happy had they been let alone. But no—they must tell all their worries—so that people will know how foolish they are!

Emotional Control

The feelings play a tremendous part in the work of life and their results are far-reaching. Too often, we allow the feelings to govern the mind and body. Too often our moods and whimsies govern us and reflect upon others. We should remember that the attitude of mind is the basis of self-control. Mind governs the ability to relax at will. Will follows the desires, hence we must govern the desires most carefully and see to it that we desire what is best for us. We must use the imagination to create an ideal in mind and desire ardently to attain that ideal—then *work* for it. Create ideals of love and tolerance, and fine traits will develop quickly in your character. Love is akin to tolerance in its broader sense and *is* wisdom in its highest sense. Tolerant love is a necessary quality in the attainment of both relaxation and happiness.

Hate actually stiffens every nerve and muscle. Hate contracts the brain and warps the mind. It can only be overcome in mind. Change the attitude of mind and the hatred disappears. Endeavor to overcome the hate-evil with good. Think kindly thoughts, and good thoughts, striving ardently to understand the good in the seeming evil, knowing the law will eventually readjust evil into good. Forgive as you would be forgiven.

Of course, it is easier to see the "comedy of errors" in others than in ourselves, just as it is so much easier to forgive ourselves than to forgive others. We quickly forget our own offenses to others. They probably forget as easily their offenses to us. Strive for an easy, tolerant attitude toward the blunders of others and help them, by your own graceful attitude of mind, to better efforts. There is nothing so potent or powerful as "example." In doing this you will gain a host of friends and—you will be able to relax at will.

Love and tolerance make the entire human being radiate and glow; they open up every avenue to successful living. *It is all a process of self-directed thought.* People worry too much and *think* too little. Constructive thought is half the battle; it is the open door to opportunity and the straight road to happiness. Constructive thought—together with right action—*is* success, it *is* happiness.

Learn to Relax

Lying on the back, "let go" of yourself, allow every muscle and nerve to relax thoroughly—just sink down—glad to rest.

Soft, melodious music is soothing and helpful. Even five minutes of complete relaxation, with rhythmic breathing, will readjust the entire body and give it an opportunity to become revitalized.

Test

EXERCISE 3.—Lift the right leg and foot about eighteen inches from the bed and let it drop, allowing every muscle, sinew and nerve to flop—let go! Breathe rhythmically.

Repeat with the left leg and foot. Relax the toes and feet too.

Lift the right arm and hand to an angle of forty-five degrees and let it drop, perfectly limp and helpless to your side.

Repeat with the left arm and hand. Relax the wrist and fingers also.

Now lift the head forward and allow it to drop back—absolutely relaxed.

Next relax the facial muscles; the eyes; the tongue—lie absolutely inert—quiet. Breathe softly, rhythmically, easily, and joyfully.

Test yourself repeatedly until you can relax thoroughly—at will.

Mental Attitude

The mental attitude is of paramount importance. Perfect physical relaxation cannot be attained without mental control and to the extent of permitting no thoughts or ideas of fear, worry, anxiety or alertness to possess the mind. As fast as such thoughts gain entrance they should be overcome or expelled and replaced immediately by happy, constructive thoughts. Repetition of the relaxation tests is sometimes necessary after one tiny little wrong thought has had possession of the mind for a moment. Even the slightest tenseness must be overcome completely. The "don't care" attitude of mind is a good way to relax, but better still is the complete transmutation of thought, changing fear into confidence, hate into love, anger into tolerance, and anxiety into peaceful trust in Absolute Law. In this way a balance of the "opposites" is acquired and one may tread the middle path of peace. Bodily restlessness marks our generation. When this is overcome, mental restlessness may also be overcome. It is a matter of desire for self-improvement and—will power.

Sleep

Relaxation and sleep are the perfectly natural reaction after exertion and the fatigue following the constant daily resistance of the life-force. From seven to ten hours sleep are required by the human being, varying with the age, occupation and health of the individual. People, who relax systematically while employing the Indian system in their work, exercise, or play, require less sleep than people who do not understand its scientific uses of posture, relaxation, and muscular control. Proper breathing and diet also increase the natural resistance while the mental attitude governs all. Habit is a strong factor. It is easy to be lazy and sleep too much. Time wasted in oversleeping cannot be made up. Too much sleep is enervating.

Darkness and quiet are the natural environment for restful sleep, especially for nervous people, invalids, and children.

Do not face a bright light, the sun or moon.

The hours between ten P.M. and five A.M. are the best for sleeping; the vitality is lowest at this time. If need be, sleep earlier, and later. Too little sleep does not permit the body to readjust itself to the reception or the resistance of life-force or perform the necessary chemical adjustments.

Sleep out of doors if possible and practicable. Do not fear the night air—it is full of oxygen and life—and the only air there is at night. Arrange for proper protection against cold, wind, rain, or snow. Flannelette sheets and pillow slips add to the comfort in cold weather as do flannel gown, cap, and socks. The vitality is naturally low at night and, as the major part of the blood is said to center in the small of the back, the extremities may easily feel cold. It is almost impossible to relax when thoroughly chilled. It uses up energy to keep warm. Use light-weight but sufficient covering. This is largely a matter of habit. Heavy non-porous bedding keeps the invisible gases and perspiration close to the body and tends to reabsorption, which is not healthful.

If you sleep indoors be sure to ventilate the room well, providing for a free circulation of fresh air. The room should be given a thorough air-bath before retiring, especially if a stove or lamp has been consuming the oxygen, or if people have been sitting in the room. (Their body odors and gases pervade the air). Air out all cigar or cigarette smoke; the fumes of tobacco are poisonous and the smoke injurious to the eyes and lungs.

The Indian heads north and south, to be in line with the earth's currents. If you will face west, with the setting sun upon retiring you will, in all probability, find yourself facing the rising sun in the east upon waking—if you are very normal. You may notice too that you are breathing through a different nostril! Indians attach significant meanings to these apparently minor details—but they are capable of exhibiting unusual powers.

Beware of cramped positions. Habits of posture during rest or sleep frequently prohibit free circulation and tense the nerves. When muscles are cramped or tensed, the subject is more susceptible to noise and irritating vibrations. Internal organs, cramped, twisted, or pressed upon, cannot function efficiently during sleep. The posture should be easy, on the side or back, the legs not drawn up too much and the arms not over the head. Always relax and test your relaxation. It is impossible to obtain the full benefit of sleep with inflexible muscles, a rigid spine, or tensed nerves.

Above all, avoid too strenuous mental exertion just before retiring. If you would sleep peacefully do not engage in an argument or tiresome discussion or give way to emotional excitement. Give no place in your mind to envy, malice, or any of the lower emotions. Complete cessation of all mental activity is necessary. Eradicate all sense of fear with *knowing* and thinking only of peace, happiness, love and confidence in the Father. Like the Indian, give yourself over to the care of the Perfect Protection.

The Indian has a way of going over each event of the day, mentally, just before dropping off to sleep. He allows the panorama of "his day" to unfold itself before his mental vision, in retrospect, beginning at the close and reeling off like a bit of motion-picture film to its beginning. In this way he is frequently able to revert effect to its cause and get a better understanding. It is a splendid idea, for, by correcting the thoughts and behavior, by acknowledging to oneself the mistakes of the day and by trying to realize wherein one might have done better, there is a natural, steady growth and improvement. This procedure has a marvelous effect upon the building of character and serves to draw forth potential possibilities and powers during sleep. This was also a favorite practice with the ancient Greeks; Pythagoras always required it of his pupils.

If thus we would plan how to improve upon our behavior next time, and, without worrying about it, dismiss the matter from our minds, sleep would come more easily. Turn a deaf ear to all noises that you cannot hinder without interfering with the other fellow's rights, acquire the mental attitude that they cannot disturb you, and make up your mind to sleep—that is what you went to bed for! Think peace, poise, rest, and confidence within, and—use your will power. Breathe rhythmically, keeping the body and mind thoroughly pliable and flexible. Radiate peace with each breath and send forth love and sympathy to a suffering world that needs even your little benediction.

CHAPTER VI

PRELIMINARY INSTRUCTIONS

In the Indian athletic system every movement has been carefully studied and worked out scientifically. Each motion has a definite aim and purpose; not an atom of energy is wasted. To obtain the best results it is therefore important to read the instructions over very carefully, as the method employed is entirely different from most systems of physical training.

Remember always that the great benefit lies in the *way* in which an exercise is performed rather than in the number of times it is executed. Speed is an absolute hindrance to right performance until the method is thoroughly mastered. To go through a number of exercises rapidly but incorrectly, will frequently do more harm than good; further, the exercise will fail of its purpose.

The secret of successful body development is in doing the exercises *correctly,* by bringing the right muscles into play in the right way, and by placing the emphasis of the weight where Nature intended it to be carried.

The Indian has proved that it is far more desirable to develop long flexible muscles than bulky, knotted ones. He carefully avoids any unnecessary tensing or stiffening of his muscles, for he well knows that by so doing the circulation of the blood is impaired, with consequent improper nourishment and devitalization of the body cells. For example, clench your fist hard and observe how the circulation is immediately checked. The fingers and nails soon become blue while the veins in wrist and arm enlarge from pressure! The same thing takes place when exercising with tensed muscles in any part of the body.

It is well known that muscular action is most valuable in forcing poisons and effete matter from the body, but with tensed muscles and restricted circulation, how is it possible for elimination to take place effectively? The most important glandular functions and the vigorous circulation of the blood and nerve currents can only take place when they are not inhibited.

This is particularly true of all mental messages to and from the brain through the nerves. Any tenseness or rigidity of the head or neck muscles restricts those important and delicate nerves which cross at the base of the brain at the back of the neck. Glands of the throat are frequently affected at the same time and become enlarged or injured, due to faulty posture and impaired circulation.

Be careful not to carry the shoulders, arms, head or neck in a rigid or stiff posture while walking or exercising. In fact, never tense or stiffen the body in rigid attitudes. All the joints should be kept free and limber. This may be accomplished by learning to manipulate the ligaments and muscles which control them.

It is of the greatest importance that the spine should be flexible, never rigid or deeply curved in at the small of the back. The spine of an Indian athlete, while absolutely flexible, is as supple and strong as a tiger's. The spine is composed of a column of small bones or vertebræ held together by ligaments and muscles, and so designed as to facilitate movement in any direction with the slightest effort or swaying of the body or its members. The back was never intended to be carried rigidly stiff, had it been, it would have been just one long, straight bone. A rigid spine is extremely unhealthful; tiresome to hold, and makes proper breathing difficult. It uses up energy unnecessarily and causes a prim, awkward gait. The Indians *control* the muscles that manipulate the spinal vertebræ, always keeping them perfectly limber, ready for instant action or for relaxation at will. With habits of tension the whole life tends toward contraction; no wonder the white race cannot relax! How can perfect EX-pression come with CONTRA-action?

Only when the spine is absolutely free of all tension are the small muscles, which connect the many vertebræ that form the spine, capable of being properly developed. Exercises which lengthen and strengthen these powerful little muscles and ligaments, and at the same time produce flexibility, are of tremendous importance. Their movement must be facilitated in all directions—naturally.

It is necessary also that all the other joints of the body should be kept perfectly flexible, limber and thoroughly lubricated. This can only be accomplished through proper exercise and manipulation, preferably self-performed, in a natural way.

An Indian never forces his chest up, for he knows that it will lift to its natural position when his spine, neck, head and shoulders are properly poised. He develops his chest in the natural way, by proper breathing and muscular movement while breathing.

Many of the exercises and instructions given herein are entirely different from the popular methods in vogue today, but the Indian's system has stood the test of centuries and has never been excelled. The outstanding features are flexibility of spine and joints, long, pliable muscles, naturalness with easy relaxation, and, mental coördination and self-control together with tremendous endurance.

The basic principles of the Indian's system may be applied to hundreds of exercises not given in this book and to all forms of labor.

In all corrective work it requires patience to overcome the old habits and persistence to acquire the new. Do the exercises just a few times at first and increase the number of times as your strength and ability improve. If the muscles are sore after exercising, it is merely because they have not been properly used before. Keep right on and the soreness will pass away in a short while. The ultimate results are worth every effort many times over. If you hold on with the tenacity of an Indian, you are bound to win out and realize, too, that success is its own reward.

INSTRUCTIONS

1. Before performing any exercise read the instructions over carefully at least three times, getting all the particulars thoroughly in mind.

2. Concentrate the mind upon carrying out the instructions correctly, trying to perform the exercise efficiently and endeavoring to improve with each repetition. Correct performance is essential. Do not hurry.

3. Intend the will power upon accomplishing the desired *purpose* of the exercise. The more thought you put into the work, the more you will get out of it. Action and reaction are equal. Get the full benefit of the work both mentally and physically. When the mind wanders— pull it back.

4. Energy follows thought. This is a basic principle of paramount value. Decide what you are going to think with each set of motions and then concentrate the thought and energy upon attaining a definite result.

Think health, strength, grace and beauty.

Feel happiness, rhythm, harmony and joy, poise and balance.

Appreciate life, Nature, God and their blessings.

Enjoy the work in a spirit of play; make it a pleasure.

Know power, ability, health and strength are yours by right.

Radiate love, happiness, joy and health.

Imagine yourself improving, growing, *becoming* what your ideals picture.

Realize that there are limitless possibilities if you persevere; persevere in physical endeavor, and persevere in holding a constructive mental attitude. We are what we think; we may become what we imagine, desire, and work for mentally. We are our only limitations; we are the greatest hindrance to ourselves.

5. Stretch and reach for power, strength, or whatever is greatly needed or desired, then *pull* and *draw* it toward you and into you with imagination.

6. Music is a tremendous aid in establishing rhythm when exercising, and should accompany all motor work when possible. Music should be carefully selected, however, as the lower emotions are easily aroused through syncopated jazz while the higher emotions are awakened through harmonious rhythms and melodies. Rather than "pep up" and "excite" to impulsive or thoughtless action, strive to acquire that calm and graceful poise so admired by all. Jazz irritates the nerves and disturbs the mind. The mind should be kept cool and balanced, alert but steady, for true efficiency. Indians used to excite themselves with wild dancing and irritating sounds when preparing to kill their enemies! They used only gentle rhythms in all peaceful pursuits. We sometimes wonder if Twentieth Century morals and crime are an outcome of too much jazz music and living. We should "do anything to end the kind of jazz called hot—that insane thumping and tooting, without tune, reason or melody. The real tom-tom, from which jazz was taken, is wonderful. Through its progressive rhythms, its has almost hypnotic effect. You feel the mountains begin to sway and swing. Our jazz is merely stupid noise." *

What a pity to bequeath to an unborn generation such a substitute for music. Our Twentieth Century should not be represented in musical history with anything like jazz, cacophony or any meaningless jumble of sounds for that matter; but such a deplorable reputation is sure to be ours unless changed by the youth of today with their demand for music that is melodious, harmonious and rhythmically fine.

* Harry Carr in Los Angeles "Times."

The taste for good music should be cultivated along with the wilful direction of the thoughts accompanying each exercise. From the rhythm of the heart-beat to the harmony of the spheres, all is music. Everywhere it is present, as radio has demonstrated. Without good music life is discordant. Its rhythm makes all burdens light, it changes the character and quality of the thoughts and feelings. No one can live healthfully, happily or normally without musical rhythm in his every thought and action. Fear, worry, discouragement and hatred disappear before its magic charm; it soothes pain and heals the sick, as our red brother has long demonstrated. True music stirs that spirit in man that catches inspiration.

7. Do not overstrain or overexert yourself while exercising; take the movements slowly and easily until thoroughly familiar with them. Select those exercises which will develop your body into a more perfect symmetry of form, and do each one four or more times daily. Increase the number of times as you gain strength and aptitude. If the muscles are sore at first, it is because they have not been used; the soreness will wear away if you keep right on, regardless; strength and endurance will increase slowly but surely.

Self Development

Study yourself, nude, before the mirror and observe which parts of your body are underdeveloped or out of alignment. Be quite severe in your criticism for it is human nature to believe that our bodies are quite satisfactory. It is like standing up for your car or your family. Habits of posture need careful consideration in order to make the body symmetrical.

Choose exercises suited to your own particular needs, selecting movements that will build out the hollows and reduce the humps. Develop and strengthen the small, flabby muscles and increase the flexibility of the joints. Familiarize yourself with the different types of exercises and make a varied selection, choosing movements that will exercise the entire body every day. In your zeal to develop or reduce one part of the body do not entirely neglect the other parts. The purpose of each exercise is given along with the directions.

To insure suppleness, practice getting down on the floor and getting up again, squatting, stooping, bending, etc. Middle-aged people are apt to avoid such movements and allow themselves to become stiff and awkward and thus appear old in their actions. Force yourself into all forms of activity. The ways of modern civilization are not normal; we use less than half our muscles in the ways intended—normal labor, walking, running, etc.

Exercise or work until you perspire freely thus forcing out systemic poisons through the pores of the skin. Wash off with warm water or a quick hot shower, to cleanse the pores, then follow with plenty of cold water and a good brisk rub. To slap and rub the body, massaging the sore muscles, is good exercise in itself.

Reducing

Excessive fat—that bugbear of middle-age! There is no need to have it once you have made up your mind to be rid of it. It is ugly and useless, clumsy and harmful. Excessive fat spells lack of elimination and improper assimilation; both due to such causes as sluggish glands, insufficient mastication, impure blood, lack of sunshine, improper breathing, lack of exercise, lack of cell salts and wrong mental attitudes. First, get rid of the *cause*. In nine cases out of ten faulty elimination in one form or another is the cause. Complete elimination of every sort not only reduces excessive fat but is a great factor in promoting health and long life.

Do not imagine for a moment that fat is good for you or that you are the one human in the world who cannot reduce. You can be rid of it if you *will*. But above all, do not attempt to reduce too rapidly; that is dangerous. It takes time and much energy for the blood to carry off pounds and pounds of waste tissue, and it is a slow process at best. It takes time to accumulate fat and patience to dispose of it again. Safe methods of reduction may be slow but Nature is slow— and safe.

Many exercises are given in Part II that are most helpful in reducing weight and in modifying bulging lines. Select exercises that will lengthen and pull the bulky parts. Much stretching, with twisting and turning, is beneficial, along with punching, squeezing and kneading of the pudgy fat. Soften it and it will dissolve more readily. Working the muscles burns up the flabby tissue. Try fast walking, dancing, swimming; walking or running on all fours; rolling on the floor or ground (not a soft surface) ; take vigorous stooping and bending exercises. Sun baths and sweats are splendid as are shower baths of long duration, say ten to twenty minutes over the fatty parts, followed by plenty of cold water and vigorous rubbing.

Then curb the appetite. Diet—that hated word! "Corrective eating" is a much less irritating term. Proper diet does not mean going without everything you like; it means eating in moderation the things that your body needs instead of being a slave to what you like just because it tastes good. The mental attitude has much to do with it all. Use will power. Lack of space precludes further discourse on this interesting subject.

CHAPTER VII

POSTURE AND CARRIAGE

Personality

It is human nature to judge our fellow men principally upon their personal appearance. The first impression is usually the most vital, for, through it alone, we frequently stand or fall in the eyes of the world. Personal appearance is all that man has to recommend himself until an opportunity is offered for some display of character. There is nothing more impressive than a fine physique, or a fine personal appearance. Character stands forth represented in a hundred little ways in the physical body, in the facial expressions and in behavior. Erect posture, an easy graceful carriage, and a poised gracious manner are representative of self-culture, education and self-respect.

A continual effort toward self-improvement will many times spell success in dollars and sense.

It is unfortunate but too often true that the majority of persons place small confidence in those whose personal appearance is against them. Faulty posture, slovenly dress, careless grooming, uncouth manners, and eccentric habits are naturally repugnant. Nine times out of ten these traits are taken for symbols of the character beneath. In addition to this, incorrect posture inflicts a heavy strain upon the entire organism, crowding the vital organs, restraining the free circulation of blood and nerve currents, and placing the individual far below par. As a result, irritability and ill health eventually make their appearance. But the person does not live who could not improve his personal appearance and attributes if he would. An attractive personality is largely due to persistent effort and self-education along culture lines.

A Test

If you will stand in the manner usually taught, back rigidly erect, knees, hips, and neck firm, chest held high, shoulders squared, head up and chin in, with abdomen retracted, then try to jump, you will find that you must *relax from* this strained attitude before you can make a move! This will serve to illustrate why the Indians consider the white man's posture ridiculous. Indians tell me that they cannot bear to have their children taught such an absurd posture in their schools, it is so strained, awkward and *useless*.

How Indians Stand

The Indian's posture is always flexible, easy and graceful. He does not have to relax in order to make a move for he is always *ready for instant action*. He wastes no energy in holding himself unnaturally, and no time in changing his position or muscular control for action. His carriage is natural, like that of the animals. Taking his lessons from Nature he has observed that the pliancy of the willow tree, while apparently a weakness, is in reality the key to its strength and endurance. The flexible branch bends in the gale, offering little opposition, while the stiff and sturdy branch is snapped off and destroyed by the storm, a victim to its own resistance.

Definite instructions follow, telling just how to obtain and maintain a correct posture, according to the Indian's ideal. Both his posture and carriage are scientifically adapted to weight placement, balance, complete flexibility, muscle control, and impulsions. They serve to prevent curvature of the spine, broken arches, various forms of neurasthenia, and headache, as well as many stomach and intestinal disorders. The American Indian *employs these principles of posture and carriage in all his movements at all times*. In addition he opens up certain channels that mentally control his body.

Mental Control

The effects of correct posture and carriage upon the body, nerves, and mind are of such vital importance that they can hardly be overestimated. Many valuable things are known and carefully taken into account by the Indians, though they appear to be quiet and unassuming. A discovery was made by them, or handed down from their ancestors, which is of very great value to us—the control of the physical body through the powers of mind. They are even able to control many of the so-called involuntary muscles of the body. They realized the absolute necessity of physical coördination in order to gain such control. They discovered that in order to attain any degree of mental efficiency there must be no hindrance through any of the channels that lead from the brain to the body or back again from the body to the brain. They found that the placement of head, neck, spine, nerve plexes, legs, and feet should all conform to a true and perfect alignment, with each other, and with the center of gravity. Also that this alignment—together with the weight placement, balance and carriage—should be adjusted to the center of gravity and the ground according to very exact laws. They believed that any distortion of posture, any wrong placement of weight, any lack of balance or poise, had a subtle effect upon the brain and hence upon the mind. They found, furthermore, that any inhibition to the free circulation of the blood, nerve or etheric currents in the body would immediately react upon the brain, producing mental deficiency. They believed, too, that mental processes act directly upon the body, for health or for inharmony, and in just such proportion as the aforesaid alignment or misalignment permits. Therefore, they believed that the mind cannot act with any degree of accuracy through a nervous system or brain whose functions are in any way impeded, since they are the vehicles, or instruments, for the expressions of mind in, and upon, the body.

Natural Posture

A graceful, natural and comfortable posture and an easy carriage may be acquired by following a few simple but *basic* rules. Old habits may be entirely overcome by the persistent application of correct methods.

These rules should be observed at *all times,* in every form of work, exercise, sport, relaxation, or leisure. These, together with the exercises that follow, are particularly valuable in correcting wrong posture or carriage in young children and youths. Habits of childhood form the foundation for future life.

Correct posture and balanced carriage are basic principles of the Indian system, and, while easy, require the most careful consideration and intelligent application.

The abdominal retraction of muscles should be exercised dozens of times daily until it becomes a habit to carry the muscles in and up with perfect ease. While out walking, stop occasionally to look in store windows or observe the beauties of Nature and take that opportunity to adjust your posture. Correct your carriage whenever you can make yourself think of it; that should be often until the habit is formed. Women should go without corsets and frequently practice exercises that strengthen the muscles of the abdomen, sides and back. It is not normal to depend upon a corset for support—the only sensible dependence should be upon the muscles, weight placement and carriage as intended by nature.

The Indian, like the famous Japanese Ju-Jutsu, balances his weight within the radius of a small circle. Poised in the center, with correct weight placement and alignment, he will sway to and fro and around, always keeping a perfect balance. To get off center or off balance is to lose control of himself. When wrestling, he awaits attack from his opponent and, rather than meet him with strong resistance, steps quickly aside as his adversary lunges forward, allowing him, if un-

(c)......

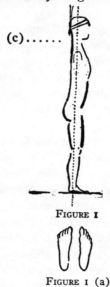

FIGURE I

FIGURE I (a)

aware of such tactics, to fall clumsily to the ground; the object being not to hurt a man so much as to cause him to injure himself.

Indian Posture

Figure I illustrates correct standing posture according to the Indian's idea. The dark lines indicate the muscles to be used and serve to demonstrate the emphasis of weight placement; the light lines indicate the muscles and joints to be kept flexible.

This posture is practiced by American Indians of all tribes who have preserved their ancient teachings. It accounts, in large measure, for their strength, agility and endurance as well as their supple grace and remarkable self-control.

Rules

EXERCISE 4.—1. Stand with the feet straight forward, placed about one or two inches apart (a).

2. Balance the weight forward, exactly between the heels and the toes, over the arches of the feet. The arch is the strongest type of architecture known, therefore the foot is so designed as to bear the weight of the entire body in the easiest and most efficient manner possible.

3. Flex the knees *slightly,* to permit of an easy spring. This relieves any jar produced by walking or jumping. Do not hold the knees stiff—keep them perfectly limber and flexible.

4. Swing the hip joints backward until you feel the weight of the torso carried well forward over the thighs. In the thigh we find the longest bone and the largest muscles in the body, designed by Nature to carry the weight and help propel the body. Be careful not to hold the hips or buttocks rigid or tensed. Keep easily poised—alert but easy, and ready for action.

5. Relax the spine all the way up and down and keep it perfectly flexible at all times. No well-trained Indian would be guilty of having a rigid spine, he knows it would prohibit freedom of movement and destroy his balance; besides it is entirely unnecessary and extremely fatiguing. Above all, be natural and never allow yourself to be strained in attitude of mind or body. Be careful *not to overdo* the posture for then you would become angular and unbalanced.

6. Draw the abdominal muscles in and up and keep them so. Get the habit. This does not mean to hold the breath. The diaphragm moves *up* and *down* quite independently of the abdominal wall. This position is much easier to maintain with a thoroughly pliable spinal column.

7. Lift the crown of the head high—"feel tall." This will draw the chin into a normal position and poise the head gracefully. Stand tall! Think right. Be clean minded, full of courage and strong.

8. Now exert a slight pressure backward at the base of the neck (c), at the hump. This will lift the chest to a normally erect position, without forcing it up, and will permit of easy breathing at the same time.

9. Flatten the shoulder blades by a slight downward movement.

10. Swing the arms and hands flexibly and freely from the shoulder joint, relaxed, but ready for instant use.

This posture insures the greatest amount of power while exerting the least amount of energy. It relieves the body from all unnecessary strain, prevents jarring and friction, is soothing to the nerves, saves the spine from shocks or wrenching, and brings untold comfort and relief.

The most perfect weight placement is thus secured by the natural system of leverage afforded by the extremely clever arrangement of bones, muscles, joints, and tendons. The long bones act as crow-bars; the ankle, knee, and hip joints as fulcrums; the tendons support the structure, while the muscles provide the medium of power. The combination insures the most perfect balance and poise, together with the greatest conservation of energy, in every form of movement in which man may engage.

Tests

1. Imagine yourself suspended by a cord from the crown of your head. The alignment will coincide, in feeling, with the line shown in Figure 1.

2. Drop a plumb line (with a spool on the end) from the chandelier or the doorway. Stand before a mirror or in such a way that your body will cast a shadow on the wall. Correct your posture by standing plumb with the line as shown in Figure 1. The line should appear to pass down *through* the body rather than straight at the back or front.

Incorrect Posture

Figure 2 illustrates the so-called "erect posture" as interpreted by many people, with the toes out as in (b). The entire body is rigid

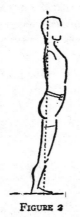

FIGURE 2   FIGURE 2 (b)

and stiff, exerting an unnecessary and trying pressure upon the spine, neck, hips, legs, and feet. It is unnatural, ugly and graceless. Owing to the intense strain of this posture it is practically impossible to hold the muscles of the abdomen in and up, and, at the same time breathe correctly. It is not natural to hold the spine rigid while holding the abdominal muscles up, nor can it be done continuously—the exertion is too great. Try it out for an hour and be convinced. It is impossible to breathe normally or comfortably in this forced attitude, or even to breathe abdominally, with the diaphragm moving in and out as some direct. Try standing in this position, rigidly erect and then attempt to make a sudden move. You will find that you must first relax yourself to a considerable degree before any movement can be made—it is impossible otherwise without straining yourself. The Indian is well aware of this fact and consequently assumes a posture that is always useful to him, one in which he is ready at any time for instantaneous action or any surprise. The Indian wisely excludes all useless movements or postures in his scientific and thoughtfully organized system of athletics.

Heels

Since normal posture requires that the weight be placed directly over the arch of the foot, it follows that the wearing of high heels would shove the weight forward upon the ball of the foot. With the body thus off balance, there is an almost unconscious effort to maintain poise by allowing the hips and abdomen to sag forward, thus causing the spine to curve in deeply at the waistline and the shoulders to become rounded while the head is thrust forward, completely out of true alignment. Nerves and nerve plexes cannot function adequately through a distorted spinal column nor can it be expected that delicate female organs could stand the pressure, strain, and pull upon their slender ligaments for long without sagging, turning or dropping. The habitual "débutante slump" tends to sag the body to one side, twisting the spine and vital organs out of place. In fact high heels really make the foot look deformed and shorten the muscles at the back of the legs until a normal shoe cannot be worn with comfort. They are a ridiculous relic of barbarism and we are glad to see that the modern young woman of brains is adopting sensible sport models and sandals. It will have much to do with making child-bearing easy.

Figure 3 illustrates the results of "erect posture" after years of
constant application. As the figure matures with advancing years, the
back sways in and the abdomen has a tendency to protrude and sag.
Many of the muscles of the internal vital organs are attached to the
spine and if the spine sways forward it is quite natural that the viscera
should sag also. This constant pull, together with the additional weight,
brings a great strain on the back and is frequently the cause of indi-
gestion, nervous troubles, backache, headache and prolapsed generative

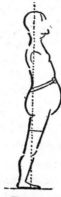

FIGURE 3

organs. It also allows the intestines to rest on or against the generative
organs causing serious displacements, foreign growths and various
diseases.

With the rigidly erect posture, the hips are forced to assume much
of the weight of the torso, frequently throwing the ball and socket
joints out of line. The feet and ankles suffer, the toes develop corns,
the knees disjoint easily and the balls of the feet become calloused.
The arches also suffer from the misplacement of weight and often
result in a faulty rocking motion of the feet in walking, especially
when one toes out. Every step brings a jar upon the spine and thence
upon the nerves and a consequent reaction upon the brain.

The restricted circulation of the blood and nerve currents is one
of the most serious faults of this posture. The body is absolutely out
of true alignment; kinesthetic control is faulty and the individual is
neither poised nor balanced. Under such conditions the brain and mind
cannot function with any degree of accuracy.

Walking

A graceful, easy carriage, especially while walking, is greatly to be admired—it is an art. The American Indian has mastered this art to perfection. He walks, runs, glides, or creeps with equal ease, maintaining perfect poise. He also moves noiselessly. Swift or slow—it makes no difference which—his method is the same.

With the increasing use of automobiles, walking seems to have gone temporarily out of fashion and with aviation, we fear, there is danger of it becoming a lost art! But only temporarily, for walking is an important and indispensable exercise as well as man's natural means of locomotion. Walking, not only once but several times a day, is necessary for the maintenance of health and happiness.

Walk whenever you can. Preferably not over the same route daily; a change of scene brings change of thought and this helps to keep one out of a rut. Make it a point to walk in the country or to take long hikes over the hills or mountainous trails for a holiday. Think cheerful, happy thoughts while enjoying the exercise. Breathe deeply and draw in an abundance of life-force to be distributed over the entire body. Walk with a free, easy, springing stride and drink in the beauties of Nature everywhere about you with appreciation.

To walk, as many do with considerable effort, pushing the foot forward and then *pulling* the weight of the entire body nearly three feet every step (Fig. 4), is hard work! With every step the weight of 150 pounds, more or less, must be hauled. If you had to pull a 150 pound weight, lifting, hauling, or pushing it at every step, you would soon realize the tremendous amount of energy uselessly expended. Walking is especially wearing when the back is held rigidly erect (Figures 5 and 6), for the jar that every step produces upon the spine is nerve racking. It produces a wobbly and graceless hip motion as well.

The Indian has figured it out so as to spare himself all unnecessary exertion and consequently can finish a sixty mile walk with perfect ease—apparently as fresh as when he started. His endurance at all times is astounding. One of the secrets is that he is never guilty of wasting energy—such as pulling his own weight needlessly.

Miles may be covered by using the Indian's system of walking and with little or no fatigue. His system is invigorating, refreshing and exhilarating.

INCORRECT WALKING POSTURE

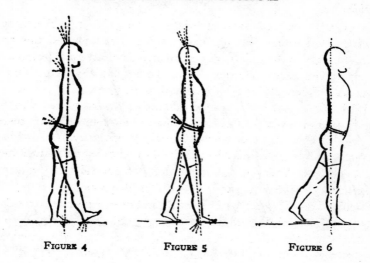

FIGURE 4   FIGURE 5   FIGURE 6

How Indians Walk

EXERCISE 5.—It is a good plan to exaggerate all of the positions and motions at first proceeding slowly and carefully figuring out the weight placement and poise.

1. Assume the correct standing posture.

2. Allow the arms and hands to hang relaxed, swinging easily and naturally with the rhythmic movement of the body.

3. Balancing on the left foot take the first step with the right foot. Use the *thigh* muscles to *lift* the right leg. Bend the knee and keep the foot and ankle relaxed. (Figure 7.)

4. The forward motion of the leg should come from the *hip joint* only. Be careful not to sway the body to one side but keep headed straight forward.

5. Swing the *body* forward. The weight of the body itself is all the force that is needed to carry you forward—no pulling is necessary. Poise lightly on the right foot as it comes to the ground, the muscles of the thigh doing the principal leg work. Balance the weight over the arch of the foot, equally distributing the burden between the ball of the foot and the heel. It depends entirely upon how fast one is moving whether the ball of the foot or the heel touches the ground first.

CORRECT WALKING POSTURE

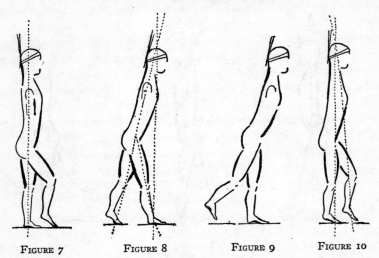

FIGURE 7   FIGURE 8   FIGURE 9   FIGURE 10

When the weight is thrown properly forward the action of the heel and toe is so swift as to appear almost simultaneous. (Figure 8.)

6. It is important that the knee and ankle should be slightly flexed and perfectly limber in order to make the step with an elastic spring and thus relieve the head and spine of all jarring. The springy motion of knees and ankles acts as a natural shock absorber.

7. In poising the weight on the left leg, when making the first step, be careful to carry the emphasis of the burden fairly distributed over the arches and thighs. The knee and ankle should be flexible to facilitate an easy, springy action. (Figure 10.)

8. The spine should be relaxed or flexible, of course, and the abdominal muscles held in and up. The head should be held easily poised, chin drawn slightly in. Any stiffness prohibits easy graceful movement. (Figure 9.)

9. Between steps an opportunity is given the free foot and ankle to take a brief rest. Simply relax them at the finish of a step and during the lift forward for the next step. When the muscles of the thigh are used to lift the leg, the knee and calf also enjoy a momentary relaxation and rest. Brief as it may be it amounts to considerable, just as the rest between heartbeats or breathing rests the organs of respiration and circulation, and gives the system greater energy and endurance.

10. Walking is a constant "falling forward," as Emerson says.

This should not be done forcefully but gently, easily, and rhythmically. This Indian method of weight placement will conserve energy and save the useless pulling and hauling of *tons* of weight per day together with the subsequent wear and tear on the nerves and muscles. Learn to store that energy and reserve it for more important purposes; to keep young and enjoy a long, useful life. (Figure 9.)

11. The breath, when walking, should be rhythmic. Practice taking the same number of steps to inhale, to hold, and to exhale. For example: Take four steps, inhaling slowly; hold for four steps; exhale slowly during four steps; hold again for four steps. Increase the number of steps to the breath as you acquire strength and power with practice. (Figure 10.)

Mental Attitude

The thoughts governing the above actions should be carefully controlled. Concentrate upon what you are doing until your muscles are trained to act as you *will*. After a while their action becomes automatic and your thoughts can be given to higher things. *Feel* light and airy, as though flying through space. *Be* buoyant and do not allow the weight to drag heavily. *Allow* only happy, cheerful thoughts to occupy your mind. If unpleasant thoughts enter your mind, banish them, or, better still, change them into constructive thoughts.

Study the action of a horse, or dog, or cat, and you will observe how gracefully and easily they move. They never allow the weight to come down with a thump. Their ankle and knee action is beautiful. This is particularly true of wild animals, they have a graceful, easy swing that domestic animals lack; partly because of confinement and partly because of cement streets and sidewalks. Mother Earth is easier to tread upon and gives much electrical energy as well. Even city-bred animals feel this and always show their natural preference when out of bondage. Mind and thought correspond very frequently with the gait. A dull, heavy motion accompanies worry, ill health, failure, and depression. A light, springy, and energetic walk will correspond to a hopeful, happy attitude; it accompanies success, health, and eagerness to get somewhere. A person's attitude upon life and his character may be read with a little study and experience in observation. Much could be written upon this subject for the play of mind upon the body and health, and visa versa, is almost endless. Think about it and study yourself, your thoughts, your postures, and your motions.

How Indians Run

EXERCISE 6.—When running, as in walking, apply the same general principles of posture and balance and the same policy, always, of allowing the weight of the body to carry you forward. (Figures 11, 12, 13, 14.)

Use the same precaution of keeping the spine limber and the abdominal muscles held in and up, to properly support the vital organs. The ankles and knees should be perfectly flexible for they act as shock absorbers, and give a springy lightness to the gait. The neck, head, and shoulders should never be held rigidly stiff but comfortably relaxed and limber. The entire torso should be able to sway rhythmically with the motions of the legs.

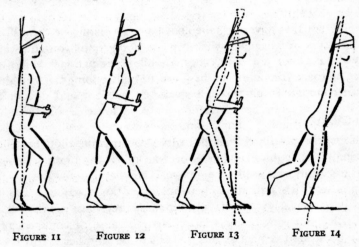

FIGURE 11   FIGURE 12   FIGURE 13   FIGURE 14

Running keeps one actively alert and stimulates quick action. It is an excellent exercise to use in developing the lungs and in testing the endurance—unless overdone; but unless practiced correctly, running may easily prove to be injurious and cause strain upon the heart and lungs. To run with a constant jarring upon the spine will eventually cause nervous trouble and sagging of the internal organs.

In running, as in all forms of exercise or movement, there is a right way and many wrong ways.

A rhythmic, rapid lope is used by the Indian for quick sprinting, while a sort of steady trot is found to be easier for long distances. Sometimes he carries the arms with elbows flexed, but more often the

Indian changes his arm position to suit his action and for relaxation on long runs. He usually carries something in each hand.

The Indian has a very graceful ankle and knee motion in running, very similar to a highly bred race horse. It facilitates alighting upon the ball of the foot and, in placing the weight forward, to "carry" the run. The balance is maintained between the thigh muscles and the tendon Achilles, the thigh pulling and the large heel tendon pushing forward, while the knees and ankles act as fulcrums. Running out of doors, on the turf or a dirt road, or, better still, upon the beach is exhilarating exercise, especially when rhythmic breathing accompanies the stride. Allow the same number of steps in taking the breath as in holding it and in exhaling again.

Stationary running is also a good stimulator. Stand in one place and go through the running motions, picking the feet up high and bringing the knee up, as close to the body as you can.

The skip or hippety-hop is also good exercise. Be very careful to obey the rules of posture and running or it might jar the head and spine, or cause the viscera to sag—especially if you do not hold the abdominal muscles in and up as you should.

Hill Climbing

EXERCISE 7.—On a hike it is advisable to wear as little clothing as you can. Wear light-weight woolens in cold weather, with soft woolen hose and comfortably loose, soft shoes. Stiff shoes do not permit one to cling with the toes or get a grip or purchase when climbing on a steep slope or over rocks. Climbing is an excellent and perfectly natural exercise, and it is always well to take a natural form of exercise, especially out of doors, whenever you can.

Observe the rules for posture when climbing up hill, allowing the weight to swing well forward, rather than pull it up, after you take a step. Allow the legs to do the work and with as little unnecessary strain as possible. The rules for walking are exaggerated for climbing. It is more noticeable that the forward leg is pulled up by the thigh muscles while the back leg pushes the weight up, using the thigh muscles to push down and the lower leg and tendon Achilles to push up: a double action. On very steep hills or cliffs, it is well to feel with the hands for a strong place to bear the weight and to assist in the pull upward. Keep the spine well relaxed and it will enable you to cling

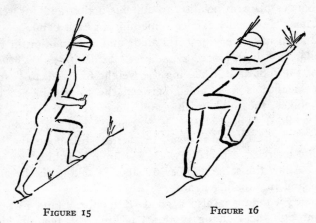

FIGURE 15   FIGURE 16

closer to the cliff and also to better keep your balance. Pulling the
weight up by the arms is always good exercise. (Figures 15, 16.)

EXERCISE 8.—Down hill the action and carriage are different in
that it is necessary to carry the weight back to prevent falling forward.
Always take the descent with flexed knees and a relaxed spine; then

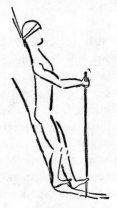

FIGURE 17

you will not feel the jar. It is necessary, on steep cliffs, to descend
heels first and, if this is done with a stiff ankle, knee, or spine, the
jar amounts to a distinct shock. (Figure 17.)

In case of falling, relax completely and you will be much more
likely to escape broken bones. Any rigidity places the arms and legs at
angles in which they are much more apt to strike a rough surface and

break. It is easier to save yourself too if there is a chance of grasping something.

Swinging

EXERCISE 9.—To the outdoor sportsman the ability to swing from branches or cliffs is often absolutely necessary. Practice swinging from tree branches, swinging the weight from branch to branch. There is nothing much better than this to limber the spine and shoulders and to strengthen the arms and back at the same time.

Allow the weight to hang by one arm and swing around to another branch, either forward or backward, and take the weight onto the other arm.

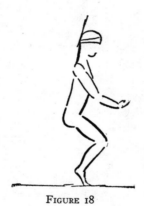

FIGURE 18

Twist the body, hanging by one arm; then, when hanging, by both arms.

Hanging by the feet, heels, or toes, and then pulling the weight up, either forward or backward, is good practice as well as strengthening.

Hang by the knees and swing, allowing the arms and shoulders to swing out, perfectly relaxed.

Many of the regulation trapeze tricks may be done from a tree, with the added advantage of being out of doors and requiring more dexterity on account of the other branches.

Jumping

EXERCISE 10.—When jumping, the Indian makes his entire body perfectly limber and relaxed, with the exception of the abdominal muscles, which he carefully draws inward and up, to form a strong protective wall to support the internal viscera and delicate generative organs. The legs are relaxed, toes pointed downward, knees and ankles flexed for the spring. This enables him to land on a cushion, the balls of the feet, and with an elastic spring of the knees and ankles that prohibits all shock when he alights. He straightens himself by lifting his weight up and forward, using the muscles of the legs. (Figure 18.)

CHAPTER VIII

HOW INDIANS USE THEIR MUSCLES

Floor and Bed Exercises

Unless you are fortunate enough to live where you can take these exercises upon the ground and thus contact the magnetic earth currents as the Indian does, the next best thing is to take them upon the floor. Many of the following exercises are excellent also to take in bed, upon waking in the morning or for invalids and convalescents. The Indian heads north and south facing the sun whenever he can.

The first thing an animal does upon waking is to *stretch,* thoroughly, all the muscles of the body. This limbers them up after the relaxation of sleep and stimulates the circulation of the blood. The observing Indian soon learned the value of this practice. Stretching is always indulged in, after any kind of relaxation, before any form of exercise is taken.

Always have plenty of fresh air circulating through the room when you exercise.

The following exercises strengthen the muscles of the abdomen, including those forming the walls which inclose the viscera, and assist the function of breathing. They also exercise the muscles of the sides and back and the muscles and ligaments which hold the internal vital organs in place.

They strengthen the muscles which support the spinal vertebræ, helping to make the spine flexible and limber as well as strong. The constant use of these small muscles in various exercises makes the spine and back extremely powerful, if properly executed.

The muscles of the arms, hands, legs, and feet are all lengthened, strengthened, and limbered into flexibility through the stretching.

These exercises are also effective in reducing excessive fat from the hips, waist and abdomen, as well as around the shoulder blades and sides.

They produce an exhilarating effect owing to the stimulated circulation of blood and nerve currents and the thorough oxygenation and vitalization of the whole body.

Remember always to breathe correctly while exercising and to go slowly at first.

EXERCISE 11.—Slow waltz music.

(a) Lying on back with the legs and arms in line with the torso:
Relax and inhale.
Stretch with both feet and both hands as far as you can reach, counting six.
Relax and exhale.
Repeat four times.
Repeat, stretching with little fingers and little toes.
Repeat, stretching with middle toes and middle fingers.
Repeat, stretching with large toes and thumbs.

(b) Same position as (a):
Relax and inhale.
Stretch with right-hand fingers and right-foot toes as far as you can reach, slowly, counting six.
Relax and exhale.
Repeat, stretching left hand and left foot.
Alternate, repeating four times.

(c) Same position as (a):
Relax and inhale.
Stretch with the right wrist at the base of the palm as though pressing hard, and with the right heel as far as you can, slowly, counting six.
Relax and exhale.
Repeat, stretching left hand and left foot in the same way.
Alternate, repeating four times.

(d) Same position as (a):
Repeat all the above exercises but *rotate* the body to the left side and stretch up and forward with the right hand and forward and down with the right foot, counting six.
Then rotate the body on to the right side, stretching the left hand and foot in the same way, counting six.
Inhale and *hold* the breath during each full rotation.
Relax and exhale.

This exercise will make the whole body limber and exercise a different set of muscles.

(e) Lying on back with arms at sides:

Clasp the thumbs and *stretch* the hands and fingers as far above the head as you can and—at the same time—

Cross the feet and stretch the toes, counting six.

Rotate from side to side, holding the breath for one complete rotation.

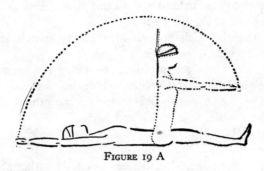

FIGURE 19 A

EXERCISE 12.—Waltz music. This exercise will bring a different set of small muscles into play and develop strength in the back, sides, arms, and legs.

Lying on the stomach with arms at sides:

Relax and inhale.

Repeat exercises (a), (b), (c), (d), and (e) of Exercise 11 in this position. Be sure to turn the head occasionally, exercising both sides.

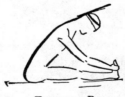

FIGURE 19 B

EXERCISE 13.—Waltz music. This exercise will limber and develop strength in the spine, hips, shoulder joints and shoulder blades, as well as the sides of the torso and the backs of the legs.

Lying on the back, feet together and arms above head in line with the torso:

Relax and inhale.

Lift the body to a sitting position, reaching upward and forward, stretching with the fingers, counting six. (Figure 19 A.)

Bend forward at the *hip joint* (not the waist), stretch forward and grasp the feet with the hands, allowing the head to bend forward. Keep the spine relaxed and the muscles of the abdomen in and up. Count three. Exhale as you bend forward. (Figure 19 B.)

Push out the back and shoulders as you pull and straighten the knees. Count three.

Swing back slowly to position, stretching the hands in an arc.

Relax and take a full breath before the next exercise.

EXERCISE 14.—Waltz music. This exercise strengthens the muscles of the abdomen, spine, legs, arms and back.

(a) Lying on back, hands clasped at back of neck:
Inhale slowly, keeping the body relaxed.
Lift the right leg, stretch, toes pointed as though reaching as far up and out as you can, and bring the leg slowly to a position at right angles to the body. Count six.
Exhale slowly while swinging the leg to position, stretching vigorously all the way, from hip joint to toes.
Relax.
Repeat with the left leg.

(b) Alternate.

(c) Alternate, stretching with the fingers and arms, upward and outward at the same time.

(d) Repeat (a), lifting the right leg and stretching with the heel. Repeat with the left leg.

(e) Alternate, stretching with the palms and wrists at the same time.

(f) Repeat, lifting both legs and stretch with the toes.

(g) Repeat, lifting both legs and stretching with the heels.

(h) Repeat, lifting both hands above the head on a line with the torso and stretching first with toes and fingers and then with heels and palms.

EXERCISE 15.—Waltz music. The bicycle tread. This exercise is excellent for limbering the joints and develops the muscles of the legs, abdomen, and back.

(a) Lying on back with hands clasped at back of neck:
Relax and inhale.
Lift the right leg, stretching as far as you can with the toes

pointed, and swing slowly in a circle, as though riding a bicycle backward. Count twelve.

Relax and exhale.

Repeat with the left leg.

(b) Alternate, working slowly and keeping the spine flexible and stretching vigorously. Feel the pull in the abdomen and back.

(c) Repeat, but with a reverse circular motion, as though riding a bicycle forward.

(d) Alternate, breathing rhythmically and slowly, inhaling between each complete revolution of the legs and exhaling at the finish. Relax.

(e) Repeat, stretching with the heels.

EXERCISE 16.—Waltz music. A good exercise for limbering the hip joints and strengthening the muscles of sides, back, and legs.

(a) Lie on the left side, left hand under the neck, right hand on right hip.

Relax and inhale.

Swing the right leg in a complete circle, toes pointed and stretching. Count six.

Relax and exhale.

Reverse the circle.

(b) Repeat, lying on the right side and swing the left leg in a circle.

Repeat, reversing the circle.

EXERCISE 17.—Music in march time. An effective exercise for strengthening the muscles of the abdomen, back and legs; also limbers the knee joints and aids evacuation.

(a) Lying on back, hands clasped at back of neck:

Relax and inhale.

Draw right knee up to the body, using the thigh muscles and pulling hard, as though a weight was tied to the foot. Count four.

Kick hard, straight out.

Swing back to position.

Relax and exhale.

Repeat, using the left leg.

(b) Alternate, kicking with force, first with the right and then with the left foot.

EXERCISE 18.—Waltz music. This exercise is valuable as a bowel
massage; it also limbers the knee joints.

> Lying on back, hands at sides:
> Relax, take a deep breath and hold.
> Draw right knee up close to the body, clasp knee with both
> hands and rotate the whole leg in a circle, three times. Count
> nine. (Figure 20.)
> Churn the abdomen vigorously.
> Swing to position; relax and exhale.
> Repeat with the left knee.

EXERCISE 19.—Music in swinging rhythm. This is a good hip reducer
and also strengthens the backs of the legs and the spine.

> Lying on back, arms at right angles to the body, palms flat:
> Relax and inhale.
> Stretch right leg, toes pointed, and raise it to a vertical position.
> Count four.

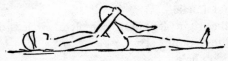

FIGURE 20

> Swing to left and touch the floor just beyond the left hand,
> keeping the leg straight and stretching hard. Count four.
> Rotate the body on the left hip as you swing the right leg.
> Swing slowly back to position, stretching out all the way, count-
> ing four.
> Relax and exhale.

EXERCISE 20.—This exercise produces flexibility, limbers the joints
and develops the muscles on the insides of the legs.

> (a) Lying on the back, arms at sides, palms down:
> Relax.
> Lift both legs slowly, stretching vigorously, to a vertical posi-
> tion, keeping the knees straight; stretch with the toes and
> fingers.
> (b) Inhale slowly as you swing both arms, stretching and reaching,
> in an arc on the floor until in line with the torso. Count six.
> (c) Now spread the legs as wide apart as you can, stretching with
> the toes. Count three. The weight of the legs will help the
> spread.

Swing back to perpendicular position, arms at sides.
Exhale and relax.

(d) Repeat, stretching with palms and heels.

Exercise 21.—This exercise will develop the neck, chest and abdomen.

(a) Lying on the back with a large pillow under the shoulders, feet together, hands at sides, palms in:

Relax and inhale.

Stretch the head and neck backward, lifting the chin. Count three. Keep the shoulders flat on the pillow and the spine perfectly flexible. (Figure 21.)

Now stretch and pull from the crown of the head, and lift the head, pulling the chin in toward the chest. Count three; hold three.

Stretch slowly back to position, counting three, exhaling.

Repeat four times.

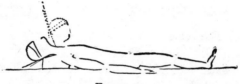

FIGURE 21

(b) Repeat, stretching the fingers and arms down at the same time.

(c) Repeat, stretching the head to the right, vertically; to the left, vertically.

(d) Repeat, without pillow. Lift head and look at toes. Stretch toes toward you at the same time: arms relaxed.

Exercise 22.—Music ¾ time. This exercise makes the shoulder joints flexible and stimulates the action of the liver.

(a) Lying on the left side, left hand under the neck, right hand relaxed on the breast, legs and feet relaxed, head on a pillow:

Rotate the shoulder joint, moving it up and *forward,* down, back and around, in a circle, pulling and stretching out from the socket as far as you can, quite vigorously. Count six.

Repeat four times, breathing rhythmically.

(b) Reverse the rotation, back and around.

(c) Turn on the right side and rotate the left shoulder in the same way.

(d) Churn the sides with the hands, in the entire region of the liver (right) and spleen (left).

EXERCISE 23.—This exercise will stimulate the circulation in the intestines and assist in moving the bowels.

Lying on the back without a pillow, flatten the spine against the floor; hips relaxed:

Relax and breathe softly and rhythmically.

Draw the knees up, keeping the feet flat upon the floor.

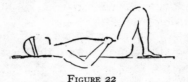

FIGURE 22

Now massage the entire abdomen, using the fists or kneading deep with the fingers, one full minute at a time. (Figure 22.)

Complete the exercise with a full breath and relax.

Foot and Wrist Exercises

EXERCISE 24.—Music, waltz or fox trot.

(a) Lying on back, feet together, hands clasped at back of the neck:

Relax and inhale.

Lift right leg to an angle of about forty-five degrees.

Point the toes and turn the *foot* to the right, down and around in a circle, stretching vigorously. Count six. Use the muscles of the foot and ankle only. Resume position while exhaling. Count six.

Repeat with the left foot.

(b) Repeat, stretching with the *heels* instead of the toes.

(c) Repeat position but *twist* the whole leg to the right, holding it upright. Repeat with the left leg. Then repeat with each leg twisting to the left, counting six for each.

Twist both *inward*. Repeat in a wavy motion, four times.

EXERCISE 25.—Music ¾ time.

(a) Lying on back, feet together, arms at sides:

Relax and inhale.

Lift the right arm to an angle of about forty-five degrees.

Point the fingers and turn the hand to the right, down and around in a circle, stretching vigorously. Count six. Be careful that the motion is made with the muscles of the wrist and hand, principally.

Resume position while exhaling. Count six.

Repeat with the left hand and arm.

(b) Repeat position but *twist* the whole arm, holding it upright, counting six. Repeat with the left arm and hand, twisting to the left.

Repeat, using both arms, twisting in and then out, in a wavy, rhythmic motion, slowly, stretching while you twist.

EXERCISE 26.—Music ¾ time.

Repeat position. Repeat exercises (a) and (b), but use the right leg and the left arm.

Repeat, using left leg and left arm, then left leg and right arm.

Repeat, using both legs and arms.

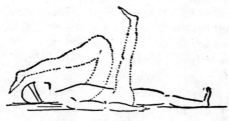

FIGURE 23

Repeat all exercises stretching with the palms and heels.

Repeat all exercises *pulling* on the return, after stretching.

EXERCISE 27.—Music, anything inspiring. This exercise is an excellent one for the spine, legs and internal organs.

(a) Lying on the floor, arms at sides: (Figure 23.)

Inhale and hold. Lift the legs straight up and over head in an arc, trying to touch the floor back of the head and shoulders with the toes, counting eight. This may require considerable practice and should be taken easily and without undue strain.

Brace the body with the hands flat on the floor.

Swing to position slowly, exhaling.

Repeat four times.

(b) Repeat (a) and after touching the floor with the toes, back of the head, swing the legs in an upward arc, bracing the body with elbows and hands, on the floor. (Figure 23.)

EXERCISE 28.—Inspiring music.

Lying on the floor, hands at sides:

Inhale and hold.

Lift the legs in an arc and when perpendicular to the body lift the body also until resting on the shoulders. Brace with the arms and hands on the floor.

When perfectly steady, stretch up with the feet and toes.

Resume floor posture, exhaling, and swinging slowly back to position.

This exercise may be varied by changing the arm position and clasping the hands back of the neck or across the chest.

EXERCISE 29.—Inspiring music.

Lying on the floor, hands at sides:

Inhale and hold.

Swing the legs up, over and back, touch the floor and then, quickly placing the hands on the floor, back of the shoulders and head, to assist in pushing the weight of the body over, carry the weight on to the feet and up to a standing position.

Many acrobatic feats may be accomplished through elaboration of this exercise. If properly done, it is an excellent way to keep limber. Children learn to do these exercises easily and enjoy them immensely.

EXERCISE 30.—Waltz music. This exercise is particularly strengthening to the spine and the muscles of the back, legs, and arms. It also strengthens the hips, elbows, and shoulders.

(a) Lying on the floor, face down, hands at sides:

Inhale and place hands palms down on the floor, on a level with the shoulders, elbows bent.

Lift the body from the floor, bracing with the toes and hands.

Slowly lift the hips as high as you can. (Figure 24.) Count six.

Slowly lower the body to the floor, exhaling at finish. Rest.

Repeat four times.

(b) Repeat (a) and when the body is lifted about a foot from the floor sway the hips to the right as far as you can and then to the left and back to position.

Repeat four times.

EXERCISE 31.—Waltz music. This exercise is good to strengthen the spine, back, legs, and arms, while limbering the hip joints at the same time.

Lying on the floor, face down, hands at sides:

Inhale and place the hands, palms down, on the floor on a level with the shoulders, elbows bent. (Figure 24.)

Lift the body from the floor, bracing with hands and feet. Count six.

Swing the hips in a circular motion, to the right, forward, left, and around. (Figure 25.) Count six.

Exhale and slowly lower the body to the floor.

Repeat four times.

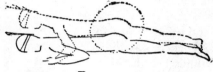

FIGURE 24-25

EXERCISE 32.—Repeat exercise 31, lying on the back with knees drawn up and feet flat on the floor. Brace with the hands, palms down, and elbows bent.

EXERCISE 33.—Music, a slow melody. The knee-chest position. This exercise is an important one and should be taken once or twice daily. It relieves all strain on the muscles which support the internal organs and gives them an opportunity to rest and regain their elasticity. It

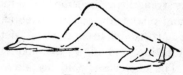

FIGURE 26

also relieves any organs of the weight and pressure of other organs which may have sagged and rest upon them, prohibiting normal function.

Lying on the floor, face down, hands at sides:

Draw arms up to a level with the shoulders and place them palms down upon the floor to bear the weight of the torso.

Draw the knees up toward the hips, lifting the torso; elevate the hips as high as you can raise them. (Figure 26.)

Inhale deeply, drawing the muscles of the abdomen in and up
and extend the ribs at the sides with the indrawn breath.
Pull, inwardly, giving the internal organs an upward lift.

Exhale slowly, relaxing all the muscles.

Repeat with each breath for five minutes.

Resume prone position upon the floor and rest, perfectly relaxed.

EXERCISE 34.—Slow rhythmic music.

Repeat exercise 33, and lift the body up from the floor, using
the hands and feet. Stretch and arch the back upward, rising
on the toes and straightening the legs.

Repeat several times before resting on the floor in the knee-chest
position. Then repeat the whole exercise after a short rest
with rhythmic breathing.

EXERCISE 35.—Music, a slow melody. The prone-hang position. This
exercise is an excellent one for the strengthening and replacing of

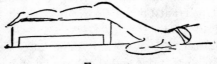

FIGURE 27

prolapsed internal organs. It permits the organs to rest and gives the
muscles which support them an opportunity to shorten and regain
their elasticity. It strengthens the supporting muscles of the viscera,
back, and spine and relaxes the spinal vertebræ, giving the cushions
between them an opportunity to be relieved of the constant pressure
from standing or sitting, and allows the blood and nerve currents to
circulate freely. The exercise should be taken several times a day
by all sufferers of prolapsed internal organs and always at night
before retiring.

Select a couch or low bed, place a small flat pillow on the floor
for your head and keep a watch or clock near. Five minutes at a time
is sufficient with rest periods between.

(a) Lie face down on the edge of the couch and draw yourself
forward onto the floor, with the hands, until your hips rest
on the edge of the couch.

Rest the shoulders on the floor, hands under the chest, palms
down. (Figure 27.)

Breathe deeply, drawing the muscles of the abdomen in and up with considerable power. Feel the pull way up inside. Feel the air fill the lungs at the sides, stretching the ribs out sideways so that the organs will have more room to move up into their normal positions.

Repeat with each breath and breathe rhythmically, counting: Four counts to inhale, four counts to hold, and four to exhale.

This exercise should be done in bed just before going to sleep and without *standing* or *sitting* up again. Give the organs a chance to stay in their new or normal position without falling back.

(b) Assume the prone-hang position as in (a).

Inhale and lift the body up with the hands, stretching the neck at the same time, head face front. Count four.

Hold for a second, being sure that the spine is flexible and not curved in "sway-back" fashion. The action should come from the hip joints, and the legs should not be stiff.

Lower the body slowly and exhale. Repeat four times.

Exercise 36.—Music in 2/4 time.

(a) Assume the prone-hang position.

Inhale and reach obliquely forward with the right hand, stretching with fingers, counting four.

At the same time stretch obliquely out and back with the right foot.

Feel the pull up the side in the entire length of the body back and front.

Exhale and back to position.

Relax and take a full breath and exhale.

(b) Repeat, stretching with the left hand and foot.

Relax for a full breath.

Alternate right and then left four times, stretching slowly but vigorously.

(c) Repeat, rotating the entire body, first stretching on one side and then on the other. Stretch with the fingers and toes one time and with the heels and palms the next.

Breathe rhythmically and remember always to relax for one full breath between movements.

EXERCISE 37.—Music in march time. This exercise is good for nearly everyone, as it gives the internal organs and the spine a complete change of position and a rest from the constant downward pressure of the upright position. It gives the supporting muscles of the internal organs an opportunity to regain their elasticity and to shrink to normal size. The blood and nerve circulations are immensely increased and all pressure from prolapsed organs is relieved.

Assume the knee-chest position as directed in exercise 33.

Lift the torso, supporting the body equally between hands and feet, in an arch. Keep the spine relaxed and walk about. Do not feel any strain in the spine or neck, hold them gracefully and easily.

Take ten steps, then stop and rest a moment. After a little practice you will be able to take a fairly long walk in this position. Walk and breathe rhythmically with the music.

Learn to trot, run, and even pace, using the arm and foot of the right side at the same time.

Children have great fun doing these exercises. Grown-ups will find that it not only revitalizes them but keeps them much younger and agile.

Scrubbing floors, polishing floors, or doing any kind of work in the all-four position is good exercise. It is too often looked down upon and too little appreciated from a health standpoint.

EXERCISE 38.—Music, waltz or fox trot. This exercise is designed to employ muscles which are ordinarily little used. It should be taken daily.

Standing on all fours, inhale and hold. (Keep the spine flexible and the muscles of the abdomen in and up.)

Balance the weight on the left foot and both hands.

Stretch the right leg out and up, backward, stretching with the toes, counting six.

Resume position (all fours still) and exhale.

Repeat with the left leg, balancing on the right and both hands.

Repeat, stretching with the heels.

Repeat, kicking.

Repeat, alternating and hopping on the foot which carries the weight.

EXERCISE 39.—Music ¾ time. This exercise is to limber the muscles and vertebræ of the neck and upper part of the spine. It will relieve the pressure on the cushions between the vertebræ and promote the blood and nerve circulatory currents. The muscles of the neck and shoulders and the back of the head are all brought into play in an unusual way, and the muscles of the throat strengthened. It will also promote glandular function.

> Lying on a couch or bed, flat on the back, allowing the head to extend beyond the edge, and to hang back and down perfectly relaxed, hands at sides or crossed on stomach:
>
> Inhale slowly and hold.
>
> Stretch the head out and upward, slowly pulling it forward and drawing the chin in to the throat. Count six. Feel the pull from the crown of the head, as though you were being pulled by a string, upward. Keep the body quietly flexible—not stiff.
>
> Exhale slowly and allow the head to relax and hang.
>
> Repeat several times.

EXERCISE 40.—This exercise will relieve tension in the back of the neck and all pressure on the cushions between the vertebræ and allow free circulation of the blood and nerve currents; it will also promote glandular function and mental control.

> Lying on the couch face down, hands at sides, body flexible, relaxed:
>
> Allow the head to extend over and beyond the edge of the couch and hang perfectly limp and relaxed.
>
> Massage the back of the neck with the fingers and manipulate all the muscles from the bony part of the back of the head as far down the back and shoulders as you can reach. This will frequently relieve gas pressure in the stomach or intestines.

EXERCISE 41.—Same position as in exercise 40.

> Inhale and hold.
>
> Lift the head and stretch the chin up, forward and back as far as you can. Count six.
>
> Pull up and forward from the crown of the head, stretching all the muscles of the back of the neck, and draw the chin in, toward the throat. Count six.
>
> Exhale and relax the head, allowing it to *drop down* and *forward*. This sudden drop will help to allow the vertebræ to align themselves normally, the weight of the head doing it naturally and without injury.

Repeat several times, increasing the number of times as you
grow stronger and gain control.

Repeat, stretching the head and neck obliquely up to the right
and *pull* from the crown of the head obliquely down to the
right.

Repeat, stretching the head and neck obliquely up to the left
and pull from the crown of the head obliquely down to the
left.

Repeat, stretching the head obliquely up to the right and pull
obliquely down to the left; and vice versa.

EXERCISE 42.—Music 4/4 time. This exercise is a splendid spine
stretcher and lubricator. It relieves spinal pressure and releases the
cushions, the shoulder sockets, the hips, and feet. It promotes the
various circulations of the body and stimulates the liver and gall.

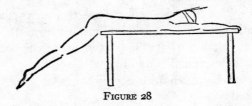

FIGURE 28

(a) Lie prone upon a table, face down, grasping the upper edge of
the table firmly with both hands. Relax the body thoroughly.
Breathe rhythmically and quietly, without effort.

Slide back and down until the body is thoroughly stretched and
the weight of the hips and legs have a decided pull upon the
spine. Count twenty. (Figure 28.)

Pull the body forward, using the muscles of the arms and hands.
Repeat several times.

(b) Position the same as (a).

Allow the body to slide down as far as you can and inhale;
then—

Lift the right leg out and back, stretching with the toes and
rotating the body a little to the left side, stretching the right
side.

Exhale slowly while rotating back to position.

Repeat with the left leg, stretching and rotating.

CHAPTER IX

HOW INDIANS SIT

The same basic principles for posture are employed for sitting as for standing. The Indian, when living a natural outdoor existence, makes use of several sitting postures which the white man has little opportunity to employ in civilized life, but which are excellent practice for development and poise and are of great value when vacationing in the big out-of-doors. A brief outline will suffice.

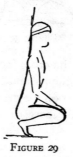

FIGURE 29

All Indian postures are studied; they are absolutely balanced, natural and easeful. Whether on the ground, a log or a rock, the Indian sits ready to spring into instant action—and this without any tenseness of the muscles or nerves. Even when crouching, he half squats with the weight well forward, but still poised, so as to lift himself instantly, using the thigh muscles for the pull and the tendon Achilles to push himself up. (Figure 29.)

When mounted upon his pony, the Indian again employs his thigh muscles to bear his weight. His legs and feet either hang relaxed or hug the pony. His spine is always relaxed or at least absolutely flexible. His abdominal muscles hold the internal vital organs firmly in place as a precaution against misplacement through jolting.

Hygienic Posture

The unquestionable value of a helpful posture when evacuating the bowels has long been understood by the Indian, therefore he squats,

with the knees well up so that the muscles may easily push forth the
feces. This position helps to open and relax the anus. (A hassock or
box will answer the purpose in the bathroom, to rest the feet upon
and help to force the knees up while at stool.) The Indian method,
however, is the natural and normal way.

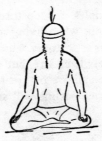

FIGURE 30

At meal time the Indian sits cross-legged upon the ground with his
weight well forward on the thighs and legs and the tip of the coccyx
(the extreme end of the spine) on the ground. (Figure 30.) He believes
that the nerve ganglion at the base of the spine is sensitive to earth
currents from which he draws power, as do animals, plants and trees;
he also contacts electricity from earth and air; he is grounded. Sitting

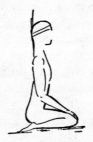

FIGURE 31

thus he can easily sense earth vibrations such as hoof beats and can
thus be warned of an approaching enemy.

As a rule, the Indian kneels or squats upon the ground while
employed in his arts and crafts or when cooking. In all cases the torso
is always poised well forward, the thighs assuming the burden of
the weight. (Figures 29 and 31.)

If you will try out some of these natural postures while sitting at your work, you will find them both helpful and restful besides keeping the knees and ankle joints limber. The author finds that sitting cross-legged on a couch or the ground while writing is by far the most comfortable attitude and much less fatiguing. The alignment of spinal vertebræ, nerves, neck, head, and brain all work together better for normal mental efficiency. Until taught to sit on chairs, children invariably prefer the ground or floor even when quite grown up.

The Indian seer or adept, who must not be confounded with the ordinary fakir or commoner type of Medicine man, meditates and thinks upon his God and the universe in this or a similar position. (Figure 30.) Sometimes he places a heel against the anus, to close it, thus preventing the influx of lower forces. He keeps his vital energies and nerve currents circulating within his body, in the form of an eight, and in some cases a double eight, while keeping the mind positively receptive to higher forces from the sun and the universal mind of Manitou. In this way he maintains perfect mental control over his entire body and his emotions. This posture is accompanied by a controlled, rhythmic breathing which produces (with meditation, thought and pure living) some very remarkable powers. *Only prepared disciples are trained after they prove that they are ready for the work.* Their methods are similar to the higher Hindu *Raja* Yoga practices. Both are guarded with great secrecy, it being considered very dangerous to play with the inner hidden fires and powers of man without due preparation and a purely unselfish desire to live and work for humanity. Otherwise, they believe, dark forces or evil entities may intrude and even take possession of the body. They also believe that such is the case with insanity—some entity having taken possession of a living body while the mind of the rightful occupant was not in full control. Many cases of obsession are of a like nature, but are removed with proper treatment of an occult nature with which the Indian seers are perfectly familiar.

Sitting Posture

To assume the correct sitting posture may seem a bit difficult at first, especially if old habits of sitting have twisted the body out of true alignment. When the correct posture is habitually employed one may work with much greater efficiency of body and with a minimum of fatigue, both physically and mentally. (Figure 32.)

Rules

EXERCISE 43.—Select a straight chair, one which is deep enough to accommodate the length of your thigh, and at the same time high enough to permit your feet to rest on the floor comfortably but not force your knees up.

(1) Sit as far at the back of the chair as you can, with the hips well up against the back of the chair—so far back that you feel almost as though you were going to sit on the back of the chair. This will serve to throw the emphasis of the weight of the entire body well forward upon the thigh muscles. The thigh is designed to do just such heavy work, having the longest bone and the largest muscles in the body.

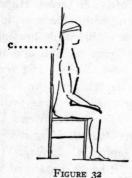

FIGURE 32

Test your weight placement on the thighs by swinging the feet and by swaying the body in a circular motion from the hip joints. Keep the weight forward.

(2) Relax the spine completely. This will also tend to relax the arms, shoulders, chest and neck. Now relax the legs from the knee and the feet.

(3) Draw the abdominal muscles inward and up. This can only be done properly with a relaxed spinal column. Breathe naturally from the diaphragm, allowing the muscles to move *up and down*. This will retract the abdominal walls and lift the weight of the viscera from the spine. It will also serve to normalize any extreme hollow in the small of the back.

(4) Press back at the "hump" of the neck (c). This will lift the chest to an easy and normal position without strain, and will poise the head gracefully. Draw the chin in gently.

(5) Flatten the shoulder blades by a slight backward and downward pressure. Do this without rigidity or stiffness; remain perfectly flexible.

(6) Feel as though you are drawn upward from the crown of your head and as though you are "sitting tall." Alignment is from the top of the head, thence through the hump of the back of the neck and down the spine.

(7) Be sure to tilt the body forward enough so that the tip of the coccyx rests on the seat of the chair, not bent under or resting on its curve.

Figure 33 illustrates a rigid, tense, and "erect" posture; unnatural and exhausting. The rigid spine, the forced lifting of the chest, the stiff neck and tensed muscles of the entire torso are not only useless, but injurious. The weight is placed upon the coccyx and hip

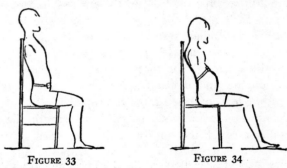

FIGURE 33   FIGURE 34

joints. This will cause undue pressure upon a delicate nerve plexus at the base of the spine, and tend to displace the hip bones. This posture is ugly and angular—it looks strained and anything but graceful. To attempt to hold a rigid posture, and at the same time hold the abdominal muscles up, makes breathing difficult and unnatural, especially if the spinal column is stiff and the breathing is abdominal.

Figure 34 illustrates the careless slump. This posture not only places the principal weight on a curved back, and the backs of the hips, but twists the sacrum and coccyx. It throws the entire spine out of alignment, prevents free circulation of the blood, impinges delicate nerves and inhibits the glandular functions. At the same time it displaces the vital organs; cramping some, twisting others and bringing undue pressure where there should be perfect freedom. The neck and head suffer extensively from impaired nerve and blood circulation, which causes cell starvation, headache, nose and throat troubles, and affects the eyes very seriously. It also causes accumulations of fat about the abdomen, hips and shoulder blades. The brain becomes sluggish, the mind and memory clouded.

Sitting Exercises

There are many valuable exercises which may be taken to advantage in a sitting posture, some of which employ different sets of muscles than when practiced standing.

Use a chair without a back, or a bench. A stool will answer if it has a broad, deep seat. It is important to place the weight upon the *thighs* in all the following exercises.

The feet should rest flat on the floor.

If a chair with a back is used sit so far back that the buttocks are poised well up against the back of the chair—almost on it.

Exercise 44.—Soft melodious music. This exercise is one of great importance in the Indian system and is for the purpose of gaining control of the thigh muscles. Correct postures and carriage can only be attained through the control of the thigh muscles. Walking, running, jumping and dancing *correctly* are absolutely dependent upon using the legs and their muscles properly.

Concentrate the mind upon gaining strength, flexibility and agility through the control of these muscles.

(a) Assume the correct sitting posture, with the hips placed well back and the weight well forward on the thighs.

Spread the knees about six or eight inches apart. Keep the feet pointed straight front and flat on the floor.

Turn the big muscles of the thigh inward, pulling them close together. Count four.

Turn the muscles and twist them outward as far as you can, counting four.

Repeat in a rhythmic, wavy motion, twisting the muscles first in and then out. Eight times. Be careful that the motion is made with the thigh muscles rather than the knees. To gain perfect control of the thigh muscles requires considerable practice.

Repeat the posture and move the thigh muscles upward, counting four.

EXERCISE 45.—Slow, swinging melody. This exercise is to make the base of the spine flexible, the hip joints limber, and serves to gain control of muscles seldom used. It will stimulate circulation, lubricate the joints and relieve nerve pressure.

(a) Assume the correct sitting posture, knees together, feet flat. Place the hands low on the hips with the thumbs pressed in so that you can feel the movement of the ball and socket joints.

Relax and inhale.

Squeeze the hip joints together, hard, pressing inward just as though you might bring them together in a strong contraction, counting six.

This requires practice and, when properly done, will draw in the base of the spine and coccyx with gentle pressure making it flexible; will stimulate blood circulation and relieve nerve pressure.

Relax and exhale. Repeat four times.

(b) Repeat exercise (a) but press the hip joints *apart*, stretching the muscles to press the joints outward. Count four.

This will cause the base of the spine and coccyx to press backward.

Repeat four times.

(c) Alternate with (a) to gain perfect control together with elasticity and perfect flexibility.

(d) Using the hips as a pivot, bend forward as far as you can. Be sure to keep the posture correct and the weight properly placed. Count six.

Bend backward as far as you can. Count six.

Bend to each side as far as you can. Count six to the right and six to the left, swinging from the extreme right to the extreme left.

Bend obliquely forward in the same way toward the right. Count six.

Bend obliquely forward in the same way toward the left. Count six.

Bend obliquely backward, right and then left in the same way.

Pivot in a circle, from the *hip joints only*, slowly, and making the arc of the circle as large as you can.

(e) Repeat all the movements of (d) and stretch up and away from the seat at the same time.

(f) Repeat all the movements of (e) and lift the shoulders as high as you can, stretching the muscles of the sides and abdomen as you pull the shoulders up. If you are bending to the right, lift the left shoulder; if bending to the left, lift the right shoulder. Then lift them together on the forward and backward bends and when rotating the entire body.

EXERCISE 46.—This exercise is for the shoulders, sides and liver.

(a) Assume the correct sitting posture, feet and knees close together. Lift the right shoulder as high as you can. Be sure that the movement is made by the shoulder muscles rather than the arm muscles. Push the shoulder down as far as you can. Repeat with the left shoulder. Count six.

Repeat, both shoulders. Now move them up and down *fast*.

Repeat, alternating, slowly at first and then fast.

Repeat, shoving the shoulders as far forward as you can; then push them back, pulling the blades of the shoulders vigorously together.

Repeat, together, then alternating.

(b) Rotate the ball at the top of the arm bone in the shoulder socket in a circle; forward, then backward. Hold the shoulder and arm quite steadily while using the muscles. Count six.

Repeat, alternating and using a rhythmic motion.

(c) Be sure first that your posture is correct.

Relax and inhale.

Press the shoulder joints *inward,* squeezing them hard. Count six. This forces a strong contraction of the muscles of the joints together, a motion they seldom enjoy. It gives elasticity.

Press the shoulder joints apart, reaching outward with the tip top of the arm at the ball. Count six.

EXERCISE 47.—Slow waltz music. This exercise strengthens and limbers the muscles of the back, sides, and arms. It is a good liver stimulator also.

(a) Assume the correct sitting posture, knees together, feet together.

Clasp hands back of neck.

Relax and inhale.

Lift the torso up, stretching the back as far as you can. Count
six.

Repeat and bend to the right. Count six.

Repeat and bend to the left. Count six.

Repeat and bend obliquely forward and swing obliquely backward, stretching the muscles of the sides, back and arms
upward and out from the hips.

(b) Repeat (a) with the arms folded in front. The pull inward
and up of the abdominal muscles at the same time with the
side and back muscles is of great value in this exercise.

Exercise 48.—Music, waltz time. This exercise will strengthen the
muscles of the back, sides, waist, abdomen, arms and legs. It is also
excellent for gaining balance and poise.

(a) Assume the correct sitting posture, keeping the weight of the
body well balanced on the thighs; feet flat on the ground,
toes straight front.

Inhale as you lift the right arm and stretch it obliquely forward and up as far as you can and at the same time allow the
weight of the body to sway onto the right thigh. Count six.

Repeat with the left arm, stretching with the fingers.

Repeat, stretching the arm to the side; to the front; up; swing
down in an arc and touch the floor.

Alternate, first with the right arm and then with the left, all
of the above motions, in a rhythmic swinging measure.

(b) Lift the right arm high above the head, stretching, and point
the right foot obliquely forward to the right, inhaling. Count
six.

Hold and stretch, counting six.

Exhale while swinging down with arm, and touch the toes with
the fingers, pivoting on the hip joint and keeping the weight
balanced on the left thigh. Count six.

Swing back to position and exhale slowly; relax completely.

Repeat with the left arm and foot.

Exercise 49.—Music ¾ time. This exercise is designed to strengthen
the ankles, arches and muscles of the legs and feet. The feet should
be bare. If cold, loose stockings may be worn.

(a) Assume the correct sitting posture, feet flat on the floor and about twelve inches apart.

Lift the right foot about twelve inches from the floor, by flexing the knee, using the muscles about the knee joint principally.

Now, using the muscles of the ankle, stretch the foot down, up, and around in a circle. Count three while stretching in each direction.

Repeat in the opposite direction. Count twelve.

Repeat with the left foot.

Alternate, stretching hard; both feet up, keeping the balance.

(b) Repeat exercise (a) stretching with the heels.

(c) Repeat position of (a) but *twist* the foot and leg to the right, then to the left. Breathe rhythmically.

Both feet together. Alternate; both to the right, then to the left, then both in and out. Keep a perfect posture and balance while working. Relax completely.

(d) Assume correct sitting posture, well back, with weight balanced well forward.

Lift the right leg by flexing the knee and slightly lift the thigh from the chair. This will necessitate bracing yourself with the left foot on the floor and placing more weight on the left thigh.

Stretch with the heel, outward. Count six.

Stretch with the toes back toward the chair, then kick hard, forward and out, using the muscles of the knee. Count six.

Swing to position and relax.

Repeat with the left foot and knee.

Repeat but stretch with the toes outward. Count six, and, with the heel back toward the chair, kick with the heel. Feel that the muscles of the knee and tendon Achilles do the work. Relax.

EXERCISE 50.—Music in a swinging rhythm.

Assume the correct sitting posture, brace the left foot on the floor and lift the right leg from the hip joint, using the thigh muscles, and keeping the knee flexed. Inhale while lifting.

Rotate the lower leg, from the knee down, right to left four times, stretching.

Exhale and swing to position.

Repeat, but rotate the leg from left to right.

Repeat both movements with the left leg.

EXERCISE 51.—This exercise is more difficult and is designed to acquire balance and to strengthen the muscles of the back and abdomen.

Assume the correct sitting posture, feet flat, and place the palms of the hands at the sides, on the seat of the chair, to brace you.

Inhale deeply.

Repeat exercise number 50 using *both* legs together. Hold the breath until you have swung the legs three times in a circle. Back to position and exhale *slowly*. The tendency is to exhale quickly and hard, but learn to control the breath.

EXERCISE 52.—This exercise is to strengthen the hands, wrists and arms and to learn to lead all arm movements with the wrist.

Assume the correct sitting posture, feet flat on the floor.

Lift the right hand, wrist leading, by flexing the elbow. Feel that you use the muscles of the elbow *joint,* principally. Allow the hand to hang gracefully relaxed.

Stretch the hand, fingers pointed down, to the left, up, right, and down again, in a circle. Count three for each direction.

Breathe rhythmically and easily.

At the finish of the circle, hold the breath and shake the hand hard, up and down and then in and out. Exhale at the finish, slowly.

Repeat with the left hand.

Repeat with both hands together, swinging them inward, then outward, in circles and shake together relaxed *downward.*

EXERCISE 53.—Music, a rhythmic melody. This exercise is designed to stimulate circulation in the bowels, promote their movement and loosen adhesions.

(a) Sit well back on a very low, straight chair or box with the feet placed firmly on a still smaller box or stool. Keep the knees together. (Figure 35.)

Double the fists like two balls and place them close together against the right side, low down.

Inhale, drawing the muscles of the abdomen inward and up at the same time.

Bend forward, squeezing the fists against the leg and press
the fists with a rotary motion, into the abdomen, working
them around forcefully.

Sway backward and forward, each time moving the fists a
little farther along to the left until the entire lower surface of
the abdomen has been covered, in all about five moves to
the left, low down.

Now place the fists an inch or so higher on the right side and
repeat the rocking and the rotary motion of the fists. Each
time the body sways against the bent legs and the hard
muscles of the thighs it presses the fists deeper into the
abdomen. Repeat still higher up, each time holding the breath
during the kneading.

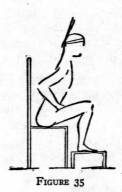

FIGURE 35

(b) In the same position as (a) repeat the same exercise but instead
of rocking the body forward and back, sway the body from
side to side, rocking forward with the swing so that the fists
press into the abdomen.

Repeat with a rotary swing of the body on the hips; swing
from the hip joints.

EXERCISE 54.—Soft melodious music. This exercise will help to
remove wrinkles and facial lines.

(a) Relax and inhale, keeping the correct sitting posture.

Relax the lower jaw and all the muscles of the face, counting
ten. Exhale while slowly relaxing and be sure to think quiet-
ing thoughts.

Repeat, opening and closing the jaw six times, slowly relaxing each time.

(b) Sit correctly but thoroughly relaxed.

Yawn, stretching the muscles with thorough enjoyment and yawn downward rather than wide. Exhale slowly through the nostrils at the finish of each yawn. Relax all the facial muscles before yawning again.

(c) Massage the face gently with the tips of the fingers, concentrating upon health, youth and happiness in your thoughts. Massage in a rhythmic rotating motion from the corners of the mouth toward the ears and toward the temples. Do not rub hard. Use a little skin food or pure cold cream to facilitate the manipulation.

Repeat, massaging from the upper lip to the tips of the ears and to the lobes.

Repeat, massaging from the nostrils to the temple hair line.

Repeat, massaging under the eyes and from the corners of the eyes over the temples to the hair, and back across the top of the head and down to the base of the neck at the back.

Repeat, massaging the forehead in circles, from the midline to the temples.

(d) Massage the neck, grasping the throat with the hand and rotating the thumb and fingers with pressure on the sides, moving them over the entire area back toward the ears while massaging.

(e) Holding the head back and the chin up, massage the neck with both hands, from the base of the throat to the tip of the chin, with alternate strokes of the hands.

(f) With both hands massage the back of the neck on both sides with the finger tips, from the shoulder blades to the skull.

EXERCISE 55.—Soft music. This exercise will manipulate the muscles of the head where it is joined to the neck, and poise the head gracefully. It will serve to lubricate the vertebræ of the neck and stimulate blood and nerve currents thus helping mental activity. It also stimulates the growth of hair.

(a) Holding the neck easily and straight without force, being careful to maintain a correct posture, pivot the head forward so that you feel the movement way up *inside* the neck where the head pivots on the end of the spine. It is here that the movement is needed rather than in the muscles of the neck. Freedom of action on this axis will relieve nervous tension and pressure in the head. Count four.

Stretch up to position, pulling from the crown of the head. Count four.

Relax the neck and drop the head backward. Count four.

Holding the neck flexible but straight, tip the head to the right. Count four. In making this motion do not bend the neck but pivot the head only.

Stretch upward slowly to position. Count four.

Repeat, pivoting the head to the left. Count four.

(b) Pivot the head, as directed in exercise (a) in a circle to the right, slowly stretching upward to position at the finish. Count four.

Repeat, circling to the left. Count four.

Alternate first to the right and then to the left.

EXERCISE 56.—Music in 2/4 time. This exercise is to demonstrate and to practice rising from a sitting to a standing posture. The object of this exercise is to place and lift the weight properly. (Ordinarily, when rising, the arms are not folded and it is easier to place one foot a trifle back of the other to balance the weight.)

Assume the correct sitting posture. Inhale.

Fold the arms; hold the breath.

Throw the weight of the body forward and draw the feet back toward the chair. Count two.

Rise slowly using the muscles of the thighs principally and press down with the tendon Achilles to force the weight of the body up. Count two.

Assume the correct standing posture, hands relaxed at sides, exhaling slowly.

Repeat the exercise five times, keeping a perfect balance.

EXERCISE 57.—This exercise is to demonstrate proper weight placement in being seated. Practice with the arms folded to acquire perfect balance. (Ordinarily the arms should hang gracefully. One foot should be a little in advance of the other.)

Stand close to a chair ready to be seated.

Assume the correct standing posture and inhale.

Balance the weight well forward, swing the hips backward and bending at the same time, let the weight of the body slowly down upon the chair, using the thigh muscles to do the principal part of the work. Keep the spine relaxed and be sure that the weight is placed upon the thighs, well forward, when sitting.

Exercise 58.—Invigorating music. This is a good exercise for lifting your own weight; it develops the muscles of the legs and back, and tests the balancing power.

Assume the correct standing position in front of a chair.

Swing the entire weight on to the left leg and foot.

Place the right foot, flat and straight front, on the seat of the chair and inhale.

Hold the breath and swing the entire weight forward on to the right foot.

Using the thigh muscles to push down, and the tendon Achilles to push the weight up, lift the body up to a standing posture on the chair.

Exhale slowly.

In descending reverse the process. Inhale and hold.

Place the weight on the left leg and foot and slowly lower the body to a standing posture on the floor on the right foot, using the muscles of the left leg to do the work. Exhale while descending.

Until you have learned to maintain a perfect balance, turn the chair sideways and steady yourself with one hand on the back of the chair.

Repeat the exercise, pulling up with the left foot and lowering with the right.

CHAPTER X

MORE EXERCISES

We will now apply the Indian system to a very common exercise, and one that is very tiring unless done correctly. Taken as an exercise, it is a splendid one and aids greatly in gaining control of the leg muscles.

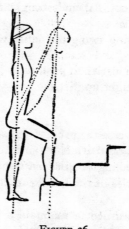

FIGURE 36

Ascending the Stairs

EXERCISE 59.—This exercise makes walking upstairs very easy. It should be practiced very slowly at first, concentrating upon learning to balance the weight carefully and using the right muscles and movements. (Figure 36.)

> Stand at the foot of the stairs ready for the climb. Assume the correct posture and inhale.
>
> Lift the right foot, using the thigh muscles as in walking, allowing the foot and ankle to hang relaxed. Place it flat, straight forward on the next step.
>
> Swing the weight forward and balance over the arch of the foot, midway between the heel and the ball of the foot.
>
> Using the thigh muscles to pull and the tendon Achilles to

push, swing the weight forward and up, pushing at the same time with the left foot with a slight spring.

Be sure to keep the right knee flexed to permit an easy spring also. Allow the weight of your own body to propel you forward.

You will notice that there is a natural tendency to hold the breath while pushing the weight upward, also to exhale with the least relaxation.

Exhale at the finish of the step, weight still on the right foot. Repeat with the left foot.

After you have mastered the ascent, the breath control may be changed to include several steps, depending upon the speed.

Next practice taking two steps at a time; then three. This is more strenuous and requires greater dexterity in weight placement and balance. It is a good exercise for overcoming constipation.

Descending the Stairs

EXERCISE 60.—

Practice going downstairs slowly, breathing rhythmically and carrying the body with grace and poise, being careful not to descend with a jar or allow the weight to fall heavily upon the heels.

Stand at the top of the stairs ready to descend; assume the correct posture and inhale.

Swing the weight to the left foot, flex the knee and lower the weight of the body, slowly, using the thigh muscles to hold and the tendon Achilles to shove the weight forward. This will naturally cause the weight to balance forward on the ball of the foot.

At the same time swing the right foot forward, relaxed and with knee bent, place it in position, foot straight front, to receive the first pressure of weight on the ball of the foot. As the weight descends fully, the flexed ankle and knee save all jar and the pressure is finally placed directly over the arch of the foot.

Exhale as you prepare to swing the left foot forward.

As in ascending, when going more rapidly one cannot breathe with each step; the breath should then be rhythmic.

Practice descending, taking two or three steps at a time; it is
good exercise and tests the poise and balance.

Exercise 61.—This exercise is to relieve pressure in the hip socket,
promote circulation, relieve nerve tension or pressure, and allow
the ball to assume its proper place in the socket. Wrong posture,
either standing or sitting, may push the ball slightly to one side or
the other and cause knee-joint troubles or arch troubles, sciatica and
other ailments. A stool will answer in place of the stairs.

(a) Stand on one step, sideways, placing the weight on the left leg
and foot.

Inhale, relax the right leg, knee and foot completely, allowing
them to hang perfectly limp. Hold the breath while swinging
the right leg freely, back and forth. Be sure that the leg
hangs from the hip joint and that the swinging motion is
done freely and from the hip joint.

To do this properly, lift the leg forward with the thigh muscles,
with flexed knee and relaxed foot and ankle. Allow the leg to
swing back by its own weight. Pull forward and allow it to
swing back again. Repeat five times. Repeat with the other
leg.

(b) Now assuming position as in (a), kick hard downward, allowing the full weight of the leg, thoroughly relaxed, to fall
downward. This completely relieves the usual upward pressure in the hip socket. Repeat five times. Repeat with the
other leg.

(c) Assume position as in (a) and repeat (a) swinging the leg back
and forth as far as you can, forcefully.

(d) Repeat swinging the leg back and forth completely relaxed,
by moving the body. Brace yourself securely with the other
foot.

(e) Standing on one foot, lift the other slightly with the thigh
muscles. With knee flexed and foot relaxed, shake it hard,
from the knee down.

(f) Repeat position as in (e) and kick from the knee joint, holding
the thigh steady.

The Swing-Hang

Exercise 62.—This exercise is designed to relieve pressure in the
shoulder joint and the spinal column as well as in the hips and knees.

A pole, tree branch or rings are the best, but a doorway casing or top of a door will answer the purpose. Any one of these must be high enough from the ground so that your feet will not touch when you hang by your hands.

(a) Inhale as you reach up to grasp the pole with your hands.

Get a firm hold, then completely relax the entire body, allowing it to hang perfectly limp.

Twist from side to side, turning as far as you can.

Exhale and stand. When dropping to the floor, alight on the balls of the feet with a slight spring, with both knees, spine and hips slightly flexed.

Many swinging and bar exercises as well as trapeze stunts are excellent when the proper postures, weight placements and balances are maintained. Follow the above suggestions for the other exercises.

(b) Hang, allowing the body to swing perfectly relaxed.

Inhale and hold.

Using the muscles of the arms only, pull the body up until your chin is level with the pole. "Chinning" is frequently done with stiff spine and legs; try keeping the body relaxed and the feet relaxed and close together.

Slowly lower the body and exhale.

Repeat several times, increasing the number of times as you gain strength.

EXERCISE 63.—Music in swinging rhythm.

Hang, allowing the body to relax.

Inhale and hold.

Using the big muscles of the legs to propel yourself, swing back and forth, being careful to keep the spine flexible—never stiff.

Exhale and drop to the ground with an easy spring, knees flexed.

In gymnasium work many knee and foot swings, and a variety of rotating movements may be added, always remembering the relaxed or flexible spine.

EXERCISE 64.—This exercise will stimulate the circulation of the blood. When cold it will warm one up quickly.

Stand correctly and inhale moderately.

Relax the entire body and shake yourself vigorously. Control the motion from the thighs, keeping the knees flexed slightly.

EXERCISE 65.—Music, waltz or swinging rhythm.

Stand correctly but with the feet about twelve inches apart, toes straight front, knees slightly flexed.

Inhale while lifting the arms, palms in, straight ahead in front on a level with the chest. Count three.

Swing the arms forcefully back, up and around in a circle and down again in front, allowing the body to swing forward from the hip joints. Allow the weight of the relaxed arms to carry the torso as low as possible and swing the arms right on through between the legs. If the swing is rapid and the arms thoroughly relaxed, their weight will carry them well through between the legs as you bend. The swing should be rhythmic as you repeat the exercise, counting six. Be sure to relax the neck and head, allowing them to hang perfectly free at the finish of the swing, and exhale with the downward movement.

Now inhale slowly as you lift the arms and the torso; at the same time stretch the hands out front and swing upward, around and back to position, in a circle, counting six.

EXERCISE 66.—This is good arm exercise and will stimulate the liver and gall while limbering up the shoulders at the same time.

(a) Assume the correct standing position, arms at sides, palms in.

Inhale deeply and lift both hands in front on a level with the chest, counting three.

Swing the arms straight out at the side and around to the back and, turning the hands, clasp them together, counting three.

Swing to the front again, as though *pulling*, counting three.

Return to position, exhaling slowly, counting three.

Repeat four times.

(b) Assume correct standing position, arms at sides.

Inhale and hold.

Hands above the head; swing them about a foot forward, counting three.

Swing them in an arc and clasp hands together at the back, low down, counting three. *Pull* to position.

Repeat four times; exhale and relax.

Repeat, clapping the hands above and below, twisting the arms
   to clap the backs of the hands on the alternate move.

Repeat four times rapidly.

Alternate all the movements of (a) and (b) swiftly.

EXERCISE 67.—Music in a swinging rhythm. This is an excellent arm
and shoulder exercise.

(a) Assume the correct standing posture, arms at sides, palms front.

Inhale and lift the arms out at the sides, palms up, stretching
   up and out, on a level with the shoulders, counting three.

Circumscribe a backward circle, feeling the pull in the shoulder
   joint. Count nine. Be careful to keep the spine, knees and
   neck flexible.

Resume position and exhale slowly.

Repeat four times.

Repeat the exercise, making a forward circle with the arms and
   hands.

(b) Assume correct standing posture, hands at sides, palms in.

Inhale and lift hands and arms out at sides, on a level with
   the shoulders. Make the pull with the wrists leading and
   counting three.

Turn the hands and wrists, stretching vigorously outward,
   palms up.

Now, with the palms of the wrists leading, *pull* the forearms
   up until the wrists almost touch the tops of the shoulders,
   counting three.

Stretch the fingers toward the neck, turn the wrists again and
   allowing them to lead, pull hard outward, with the backs of
   the hands, to a horizontal position, counting three.

Again, turn the wrists, stretching outward, turn the arms and
   allow them to descend gracefully to position, wrists always
   leading. Exhale slowly as the arms descend, counting three.

Repeat four times.

Vary the exercise by alternate moves. Pull the wrists and forearms to the shoulders three times before descending, then
   wave the arms up and down three times at the sides, wrists
   leading, in a wing-like or flying movement. This is good
   practice for control and produces graceful action as well as
   strength.

EXERCISE 68.—Music in a swinging rhythm.

Assume the correct standing posture, arms at sides, palms in.

Inhale and lift the arms out at the sides on a level with the shoulders, wrists leading.

Turn the wrists, stretching, palms up.

Swing the arms up above the head, and allow the hands to pass beyond each other in a waving motion, wrists always leading, and thence back again to the shoulder level, counting three.

Repeat three times. At the end of the third time, turn the hands, palms down, and with the wrists leading pull to position, gracefully relaxing the arms. Exhale slowly with the downward movement, counting three.

EXERCISE 69.—This exercise will limber the shoulder joints and strengthen the arms, flatten the shoulder blades and strengthen the muscles of the back. It is one of the best exercises for correcting rounded shoulders.

(a) Assume the correct standing posture, arms at sides.

Inhale slowly while lifting both hands in front, straight forward to a level with the waist line, counting three.

Stretch forward, downward and outward, and press hard with the base of the palms at the wrists. Count three.

Now swing both hands and arms outward in an arc to a level with the shoulders. Keep the elbows flexed and press hard with the wrists. Feel the outward motion of the shoulder joint and the downward flattening pressure of the shoulder blades. Count six.

Swing slowly to the front, pressing all the way back with the wrists and stretching the shoulder joint outward. Count six.

Exhale and swing to position. Repeat four times. This exercise should be repeated several times a day.

(b) Repeat the motions of exercise (a), but swing the arms up above the head, going very slowly and pressing hard all the way, and inhaling at the same time, counting nine.

Swing slowly back to position, exhaling and pressing hard.

EXERCISE 70.—This exercise is excellent for the spine, shoulders, hips, sides and abdomen. It will stimulate the liver and the circulation.

Assume the correct standing posture, hands at sides.

Inhale slowly and swing the right hand and arm back and up

above the head in a circle; bend the torso forward at the hips and twist around at the same time, swinging the right arm down toward the floor. Touch the floor with the finger tips, if you can without strain. Keep the knees flexed to avoid unnecessary strain. The left hand and arm should be swung backward and up at the same time to a verticle position, reaching with the finger tips.

Swing back to position with the same movement, describing the same arc as with the downward movement, only reversed.

Exhale and resume position.

Repeat three times. Repeat with the left arm.

EXERCISE 71.—This exercise will strengthen the back, legs, arms and arches and reduce the waist line while strengthening the muscles of the torso. It is one of the best exercises for balance and poise.

(a) Assume the correct standing position, arms at sides.

Inhale slowly while lifting the arms high above the head, stretching forward and out on the upward arc. Clasp the thumbs and reach, stretching the muscles of the entire torso. Rise on the toes and walk ten steps.

Lower the heels to the floor very slowly, and bring the arms to the sides, pressing outward, while slowly exhaling. Count three.

Repeat, running ten steps.

Repeat exercises three times each.

EXERCISE 72.—

Assume correct standing posture, arms at sides.

Inhale slowly while lifting both arms out at sides and above the head, stretching and reaching out with the fingers. Count six.

Rise on the toes, counting three.

Flex the knees and slowly squat (arms still overhead), counting six.

Rise on the toes again, counting six.

Slowly lower the arms to position as you exhale and descend to heels, counting six.

Repeat four times.

EXERCISE 73.—

Repeat exercises 71 and 72, but clasp the hands back of the head near the base of the neck.

Repeat with arms folded in front.

Repeat with arms folded in back.

Repeat with hands on hips.

Repeat with arms stretched out at the sides on a level with the shoulders, stretching outward with the fingers.

EXERCISE 74.—This exercise will limber the joints of the hips, legs, knees and base of the spine. It is excellent for poise and balance.

Assume the correct standing posture, hands at sides.

Balance the weight on the left leg and foot and inhale, counting three.

Lift the right knee as far as you can in front, and clasp it with both hands, hugging it close to your body. Count six.

Rise on the toes of the left foot, counting three.

Lower the left heel to the floor again, counting three.

Resume position, exhaling and counting three.

If rising on the toes is too strenuous at first, merely practice lifting the knees, hugging them and lowering them again; three times each, alternating and breathing rhythmically.

EXERCISE 75.—Music, waltz time, or one-step. This exercise is an unusually good one for developing the chest and breasts and to obtain balance and poise, with grace.

Assume the correct standing posture, arms at sides.

Inhale while lifting both arms in front, stretching out, on a level with the chest, counting three.

Balance the weight on the left foot, counting three.

Spring forward on to the right foot and at the same time swing both arms backward, keeping them on a level with the chest. This should be done vigorously. Count three.

Swing the arms forward again and spring back to position, counting three, exhaling.

Repeat with the left foot.

Alternate, springing on to the right foot and back, then on to the left and back, counting three for each move.

This exercise may be done quite rapidly after a little practice, and with a dance rhythm. Keep the entire body perfectly flexible, especially the spine and knees.

EXERCISE 76.—Music, waltz or one-step. This exercise will lengthen and strengthen the muscles of the back and the backs of the legs.

It stretches the spinal vertebræ apart, relieves pressure, and makes the body very supple.

Assume the correct standing posture, arms at sides.

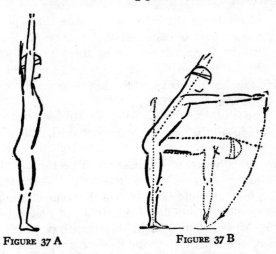

FIGURE 37 A   FIGURE 37 B

Place the feet about twelve inches apart.
Inhale and lift both arms over the head, stretching and counting three. (Figure 37 A.)

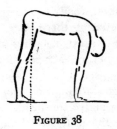

FIGURE 38

Swing the torso forward, bending at the hip joints, and swing
the hands toward the floor, exhaling and counting three. It is
not important to touch the floor, especially at first. (Figure
37 B.) Some persons have long arms and short legs and can
touch the floor easily, others cannot. Much damage and strain
have been inflicted by performing this simple exercise in the
wrong way. (Figure 38.) The real object of the exercise is
to stretch the spine and the muscles of the arms and legs.

It is of the greatest importance to keep the muscles of the abdomen held firmly inward and up while bending. If you cannot bend forward far at first, do not become discouraged; the exercise will benefit you, anyway, for it will give the cushions between the vertebræ a chance to expand and the blood to circulate through them while resting the nerves from pressure at the same time. Try each time to bend a little further, making two or three efforts with the one bend, but never strain hard.

It is advisable at first to allow the knees to spring slightly with the bend.

> Swing up and back to position, circumscribing a wide arc, stretching all the way with the fingers, inhaling, and counting six.

This exercise is practically useless when performed as shown in Figure 38. The posture is wrong, the weight placement is wrong and the hips, legs and buttocks stiff and the spine strained while the abdomen hangs flabbily and the viscera fold and drag upon the spine.

Exercise 77.—Music, waltz time. This exercise is designed to make the muscles of the waist strong and flexible, supple and graceful.

(a) Assume the correct standing posture, hands relaxed at sides.

> Bend forward as far as you can, perfectly limp, and allow the arms and hands to hang absolutely relaxed. Count three.
>
> Rotate the body to the right, pivoting at the waist line, around in a circle, swinging easily to the front, counting six.
>
> Lift to position, counting three.
>
> Repeat four times. Repeat, rotating to the left, around and up.
>
> Take a full breath before each rotation and exhale slowly while rotating.

(b) Assume the correct standing posture, arms at sides.

> Lift the right arm above the head, inhaling. Count three.
>
> Bend the body to the left, stretching up with the right hand and down with the left, as far as you can, exhaling slowly, at the finish. Count six.
>
> Repeat, stretching up with the left hand and down with the right, while bending to the right side.
>
> Repeat, alternating with a free rhythmic swing, bending the elbows.

Exercise 78.—Any rhythmic slow music. This exercise will limber the hip joints and help to lubricate the socket and will strengthen the muscles and stimulate the circulation of the blood. It will also reduce excessive fat.

(a) Assume the correct standing posture, hands on hips.

Keep the knees slightly flexed, the spine relaxed and the abdominal muscles firmly in and up; otherwise there would be considerable strain on the back and nerves. Breathe rhythmically and gently.

Rotate the hips from right to left, forward in a circular motion, feeling the ball of the hip joint rotate in its socket. Test by placing your thumbs in the joint so that you can feel the ball move about. Circumscribe a circle.

Now rotate the hips to the left, backward and around in a circle.

Rotate to the right, forward and around.

Rotate to the right, backward and around.

(b) Sway the body from side to side, moving from the hip joints only.

EXERCISE 79.—Any rhythmic slow music. This exercise is a good muscle lengthener and will limber the body generally.

Assume the correct standing posture, hands at sides.

Inhale, and at the same time—

Lift both arms straight out at the sides, level with the shoulders, turn the palms front, counting three.

Twist the entire body, from the ankles to the top of the head to the right, swinging with the arms straight out. Face as far around back on the swing as you can, holding the breath.

Swing back to the front, exhaling as the hands resume the first position at the sides. Be careful to keep the abdomen in and up, and the spine flexible.

Repeat twisting in the opposite direction, to the left.

Repeat four times. Be careful to keep a correct posture.

Repeat, with the hands stretched above the head, thumbs clasped.

EXERCISE 80.—Music, waltz or march time. This exercise will limber the shoulder joints, stimulate the action of the liver and the circulation of the blood.

(a) Assume the correct standing posture, arms at sides.

Inhale deeply and hold.

Swing the right arm forward, up and around back in a circle, from the shoulder joint. Keep the arm perfectly relaxed, the palm of the hand toward the body. Allow the weight of the arm to carry its own weight around for the most part.

Swing vigorously five times.

Relax in position and exhale slowly.

Repeat with the left arm.

(b) Alternate, first with the right and then with the left arm, with a windmill motion.

(c) Repeat (a) swinging the arms in a circle to the back, up and around.

Repeat (b) swinging to the back, up and around.

(d) Assume the correct standing posture, arms at sides.

Inhale deeply and hold.

Swing the right arm in front to the left and up around to the right, in a circle. Keep the fist folded loosely and the arm relaxed. Swing from the shoulder joint.

Repeat with the left arm.

Repeat swinging from right to left in a circle.

Repeat swinging both arms, first one and then the other.

Alternate, with a windmill motion. Spread the feet apart, keeping the toes straight front.

Repeat the above exercises with the hands relaxed.

EXERCISE 81.—Music, slow and swinging. This exercise will limber the spinal vertebræ, shoulders, hips, arms and legs.

Assume the correct standing posture, hands at sides.

Raise both hands high above the head, stretching and inhaling, counting six.

Spread the feet about eighteen inches apart.

Swing the torso forward and allow it to relax completely, bending from the hip joints as the arms come forward and down, also relaxed. Exhale slowly with this movement.

Swing the whole body from side to side, swaying the weight from one foot to the other, slowly. Relax the neck and head completely. Count six.

Swing the arms up over the head, stretching again and inhale slowly.

Resume position, swinging arms to sides as you exhale.

EXERCISE 82.—Waltz melody. This exercise is one of the most useful for everyday practice. It will develop the chest, breasts, lungs, arms, legs and torso and at the same time will greatly assist in acquiring balance and poise with grace. It is particularly beneficial for women, as it develops those muscles between the breasts and the shoulders, overcoming unsightly hollows. It also prevents the sagging of the breasts, keeps the waist slim and strengthens the back and sides. The wrists are strengthened and develop slender muscles as well

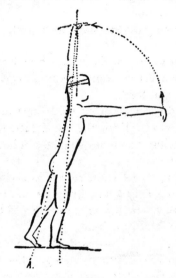

FIGURE 39 A

as the ankles, while the abdomen, if held properly, becomes almost flat.

(a) Assume the correct standing posture.

Step forward with the right foot, balancing the weight entirely on the right leg and helping to keep the balance with the toes of the left foot poised lightly on the floor.

Inhale slowly as you raise the right arm forward and up above the head, reaching forward and out, stretching the muscles all the way. Allow the back of the hand and the wrist to lead the movement. Count six. (Figure 39 A.)

The left arm should hang gracefully relaxed at the side.

Now, rising on the ball of the foot, reach up as far as you can, stretching up and backward as far as you can while holding the breath. Count six. Be careful to keep the spine and knees flexible.

Swing the right hand down and forward gracefully, allowing the palm of the wrist to lead the movement. Reach forward and pull as you swing down, feeling the pull from the palm

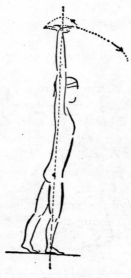

FIGURE 39 B

at the wrist joint. Count six. Exhale slowly as the arm descends. (Figure 39 B.)

Continue the pull until the hand passes the side and push back as far as you can with the palm of the hand.

Bring the hand gracefully to position.

Repeat with the left arm and hand while still balanced on the right foot, allowing the right arm to hang gracefully at the side.

Repeat swinging both arms together.

Repeat, alternating, first with the right arm, then with the left, keeping up a rhythmic motion. In this way one arm is pulling upward and the other down and back at about the same time, bringing another set of muscles into play. The breathing should be quiet and rhythmic.

(b) Assume the correct standing posture.

Repeat all the movements of (a) while balancing the weight forward on the left leg and foot.

(c) Repeat all the movements of (a) and rise on the toes. This is a splendid balancing test and uses still another set of muscles.

(d) Balance the weight on one foot, forward, and with both arms go through all the movements of (a) and (b) but instead lift them *obliquely* out and up and down. Count six up and six down.

EXERCISE 83.—Music, waltz or one-step. Develops the arms, sides, legs and ankles.

(a) Assume the correct standing posture, arms at sides.

Relax and inhale slowly, while—

Lifting the right arm out at the side, stretching out and away from the body, allowing the wrist to lead, counting three.

Swing the arm and hand above the head and over toward the left, stretching vigorously. Feel a pull in the entire right side of the body. Count three.

Rise on the toes, hold the breath and reach with the fingers, up toward the left, counting three.

Swing the arm quickly to position and relax, exhaling.

Repeat with the left arm.

(b) Repeat, using both arms and allow them to pass above the head in the upward stretch, crossing on the way. Stretch again all the way down to position.

EXERCISE 84.—

Lift the right arm above the head and stretch, keeping the left hand on the left hip. Inhale on the upward swing, counting three.

Rise on the toes, counting three.

Bend the knees and squat. Hold the breath while descending, counting three.

Rise up on the toes, counting three and stretching up with the arm.

Back to position, exhaling slowly and counting three.

Repeat with the left arm.

Repeat with both arms. This is an excellent test for balance.

EXERCISE 85.—In this exercise you may obtain considerable variety by swinging the arms obliquely up and out or by holding them straight out at the side, sometimes with the palms front and sometimes with the palms down or out. Or, twisting the arms forward and back in any of the above exercises will further lengthen and strengthen the muscles and make them supple.

Normal posture, hands at sides.

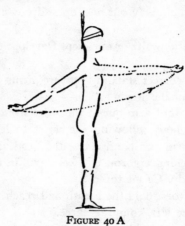

FIGURE 40 A

Inhale slowly while swinging the arms out at the sides, palms down, stretching with the fingers, and swing them above the head, palms out.

In this position rise on toes and squat, holding the breath.

Rise, stretching upward vigorously.

Swing arms to position, exhaling slowly and lowering the heels at the same time. This is a splendid test for balance and leg strength.

EXERCISE 86.—Waltz music; slow. This exercise is excellent for chest and shoulder development, also for the breasts, lungs, arms and legs. It helps one to maintain balance, gracefulness and poise. It will aid in correcting stooped shoulders.

(a) Assume the correct standing posture, arms at sides.

Inhale slowly and lift the arms in front on a level with the chest, wrists leading. Count three.

Turn the hands, palms in, and with the wrists still leading swing the arms back as far as you can, keeping them level with the shoulders. Stretch out and away from the body with the wrists still leading all the way and stretch until the shoulder-blades come close together. Count six. (Figure 40 A.)

Swing slowly to the front; count three and with the palms front and the wrists leading the way back, after a graceful turn of the hands in a flying movement.

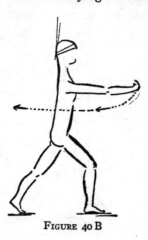

FIGURE 40 B

Again, after the palms meet, turn the hands, palms down, and with the wrists leading, swing to position, pressing out and down vigorously. Count three.

EXERCISE 87.—Slow waltz music.

Repeat the above arm movements as in Exercise 85 and at the same time step forward and swing the weight on to the right foot with the knee deeply bent, holding the balance and weight over the right thigh. Count three. Inhale slowly while going forward. (Figure 40 B.)

Swing back as you bring the hands together in front, poised for a moment but still keeping the weight poised on the left foot, and swing the right foot back, bowing deeply with the legs but holding the body and head erect and make a similar backward swing with the arms again, counting six. (Figure 40 C.)

Exhale slowly on the backward bowing motion.

Resume the original standing position, counting three.

Repeat, balancing the weight forward on the left foot and then swing back, placing the weight way back on the left foot.

When this exercise is performed with a rhythmic swing it is graceful and very beneficial. It is especially good in class work with music.

EXERCISE 88.—This exercise will lengthen the muscles of the waist and back, making both supple and strong.

Assume the correct standing posture, arms at sides.

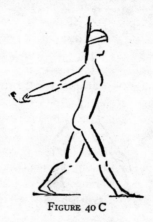

FIGURE 40 C

Inhale slowly while lifting both arms in front on a level with the chest, palms in.

Swing the entire body with the arms out, around to the right and twist as far as you can, counting six. Turn the head as far as you can at the same time. Be sure to keep the feet firmly in position and the weight correctly balanced and the spine perfectly flexible.

Swing to the front, exhaling slowly and counting three.

Resume original position, counting three.

Repeat, swinging and twisting to the left side.

Repeat, swinging to the right, then way around to the extreme left and back to position. Repeat four times.

EXERCISE 89.—Waltz music.

Assume correct standing posture, arms at sides.

Rise on the balls of the feet, inhaling slowly and counting three.

Raise both arms straight in front, palms in, and hold the breath.

Bend the knees and squat low, counting three. Twist the body from the waist up, turning to the right and then to the left, counting three with each turn.

Rise, exhale slowly and swing arms to sides.

EXERCISE 90.—This exercise will strengthen the spine, neck and waist and at the same time will flatten the shoulder blades and correct round shoulders. It will also make the hip joints more flexible and strengthen the muscles of the back and the legs.

(a) Assume the correct standing posture, hands on hips.

Inhale a full breath and hold.

Bend forward from the hip joints as far as you can, keeping the head well up, face front. Be careful to keep the spine flexible and the muscles of the abdomen drawn in and up and the knees slightly flexed throughout the exercise. Count six.

Stretch upward and swing slowly back to position; feel the pull upward from the crown of the head as you draw the chin in toward the throat. *Feel* tall. Draw yourself up and feel powerful within.

(b) Repeat (a) and rise on the toes or balls of the feet while performing the exercise. This is a good test for balance.

EXERCISE 91.—Music, fox trot or one-step. This exercise is good to limber the spine, neck, shoulders and arms. It is very beneficial to the supporting muscles of the internal organs and will stimulate the functional activity of the liver, gall and spleen. It is a good reducer as well.

Assume the correct standing posture, hands at sides.

Now spread the feet twenty or more inches apart and get a firm stance.

Inhale as you lift both hands high above the head, stretching out in front and all the way up, counting six.

Swing the body forward and down, suddenly, allowing the torso literally to fall from the hips, exhaling as you go. Allow the head, arms, shoulders and spine to hang absolutely relaxed. The knees should be flexible and active, not stiff.

Now swing the whole torso with the arms hanging pendant, forward and back as far as you can, much as an elephant swings his trunk. Repeat four times or more.

Swing back to position, inhaling as you lift. Rest a moment and take a full breath before repeating.

Repeat, swinging from side to side, swaying from the hips.

Repeat, swinging from side to side swaying from the ankles.

EXERCISE 92.—Music, waltz time. This exercise is an excellent one for general development and poise. It is particularly beneficial to fat persons, especially those with large bunches of fat around or under the shoulders and sides. It is also strengthening to the muscles of the sides, shoulders and legs.

(a) Assume the correct standing posture, hands at sides.

Inhale slowly and deeply and place hands on thighs, thumbs back, and spread the feet about twenty-four inches apart. Count three.

Lower the body to a half squatting position, keeping the weight carefully balanced on the thighs. Count three.

Now pull the right shoulder up and forward as far as you can, stretching the muscles of the right side from the tip of the shoulder to the hip. At the same time press down with the right hand on the thigh to emphasize the pull, counting six.

Relax and exhale.

Inhale and—

Repeat with the left shoulder and side while still squatting.

Exhale as you rise to position.

Repeat four times.

(b) Repeat all of the movements of (a) but, instead of pulling the shoulders up and forward, pull them up and back. This will stretch the muscles under the ribs and across the abdomen and at the same time strengthen the muscles which support the internal organs. Draw the muscles of the abdomen in and up at the same time with a strong retraction.

(c) The same movements may be gone through sitting on the edge of a low couch or stool. This is easier for most persons and a very beneficial exercise.

EXERCISE 93.—An Indian swimming stroke. This stroke is an easy, restful one to use on long distance swims and is a most perfect all-round exercise. The Indians use it frequently when they wish to swim very quietly without disturbing the water much. It develops poise and grace and may be so performed as to use nearly every muscle of the body. Once mastered, so that it becomes automatic, one can swim almost any length of time and make good headway with a minimum of fatigue—almost tirelessly.

The arm movement is made with the fingers close together and slightly bent at the knuckles or cupped on the pull.

Thrust the right hand straight ahead, palm down, and slightly turned out, cutting the water.

Swing the arm in an arc to the right, and when on a level with the shoulder, scoop it back again toward the hip, pulling hard downward; then quickly turn the hand again and pull in a powerful backward and outward sweep. It is a very full stroke and a difficult one to describe without personal illustration.

Just as the right hand reaches the hip in the downward pull, the left hand should push forward, ready for the stroke. This will necessitate a rotating motion of the body, a swaying from side to side. This acts like a corkscrew movement and weaves the body through the water with the least amount of resistance.

The leg motion may vary to suit the swimmer. It is restful to change from one stroke to another on long distance swims. I have noticed that the Indians vary in their leg stroke though most of them use a sidewise scissors kick, pulling the legs together with tremendous power.

The head may be carried in any way that suits the swimmer but probably the least resistance is met when the head rests comfortably on the water, partially submerged, making breathing easy. Be careful to keep the neck and spine flexible and *always* enjoy a moment of relaxation either with one arm or the other and with the legs between strokes. That moment is priceless, mentally and physically, and adds tremendously to the endurance.

This swimming stroke may be done on the back with good results.

CHAPTER XI

HOW INDIANS ACQUIRE POISE

In their present world-wide interest in Indians and Indian ways, the youth of today instinctively reach back toward a simpler, more balanced rhythm of life. Already tiring of their own jazzed inharmonies and the brainless rush and noise of modern civilization these clever, air-minded people are trekking for the quiet places and the Big Outdoors. Nerve-weary, fagged and half sick, we are all turning to those wise "Children of the Sun," the Indians, to teach us how to live—simply and naturally.

While physical balance and poise may be acquired, to a great extent, through corrective posture, weight placement, rhythmic breathing and exercises, real human poise comes through harmonizing the mind and soul with the various physical activities of daily life.

Dancing

"The dance cadences the soul. The history of the dance, which has often been a mode of worship, a school of morals, and which is the root of the best that is in the drama, the *best of all exercises* and that could be again the heart of our whole educational system, should be exploited, and the dancing school rescued from its present degradation. It is one of the best expressions of pure play."

Indian religious ceremonies are always accompanied by rhythmic dancing. Their most joyous festivals abound in dances and songs. The Indian is like a child in self-expression; perfectly natural.

Residents of large cities who live shut up in small rooms, with only stale air to breathe, miss many of the natural joys of life. Children, in particular, should be given an opportunity to lead more normal lives and should be permitted to do the perfectly simple and natural things that make them happy. Children love outdoor life and are naturally fond of music, unless sub-normal. Lawns, gardens and parks are ideal places to gambol and frolic. Children should be allowed to interpret music in dancing, pretending in their own way, various stories to beautiful music. It is pure, sweet play and decidedly beneficial.

Why not practice a little interpretive dancing yourself? Forget that you are grown up—be free and childlike—it will do you good and make you feel young again. Throw yourself into the game whole-heartedly. If you cannot gambol on your own or somebody else's lawn, use the radio or victrola indoors or hum a lovely melody and then endeavor to interpret in rhythmic motions what the music means to you. There is a harmony obtained thereby within the heart and soul, for it is thoroughly refreshing and vitalizing, particularly if the thoughts are kept constructively harmonious.

Indians dance for the most part on the balls of the feet, back a little toward the arch. This necessitates considerable spring at the knees and ankles to keep the balance. The ankle motion is particularly clever and is similar to the action of a thoroughbred horse—very

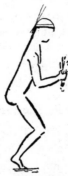

FIGURE 41

springy and light. The rise on the toes and the upward stretches are made by the muscles of the thighs, the back of the legs and the small muscles of the feet and ankles.

The spring or leap is accompanied to a great extent with the thighs and tendon Achilles and with a darting motion of the arms or body—while carrying a mental or inner sense of "flying" through the air. An Indian always lands on the balls of his feet with flexed knees and ankles and a thoroughly relaxed spine—Nature's shock absorbers.

The movements of arms, legs, feet and hands are made with graceful stretching, reaching and pulling motions in perfect rhythm with the swinging, swaying movements of the body and the breath. Every breath is timed, every move is studied and full of meaning. The weight of the body should always guide the movements by a gentle falling forward in the desired direction.

Barefoot dancing, especially in a light costume or bathing suit, out-of-doors, is very beneficial and healthful. Indians as well as many Orientals and Europeans appreciate the healing and rejuvenating qualities of the early morning dew on the grass and meadows, and eagerly absorb it through the soles of their feet while inhaling the fragrant morning air. An early morning prayer-dance in appreciation of the benefits of the rising sun is a religious rite with many tribes. In this busy twentieth-century life we do not sufficiently appreciate the tremendous benefits of Nature and the sun, furthermore we are filled with a false sense of modesty. The body should be glorified and purified and considered a temple of divinity as the Indian belief prescribes —rather than as a receptacle for the fulfillment of every manner of indiscretion and desire known to perverted man. The purification of thoughts and desires is the first step the Indian takes in the betterment of his body and his fortunes.

When practicing the dances and exercises that follow try to keep the breath rhythms synchronized with the movements of the body and the thoughts and aspirations high.

Leg Exercises

EXERCISE 94.—Music, waltz or one-step. This exercise will limber the hips and strengthen the legs and at the same time promote balance and control. It is also a good exercise to reduce the hips.

Assume the correct standing position. (Brace yourself with the left hand on the back of a chair at first, if necessary.)

Poise the weight on the left leg and foot; inhale.

Swing the right leg forward, to the right and around in a circle, reaching out with the toes as far as you can, stretching all the way.

Each time try lifting and swinging the leg a little higher up.

Resume position and exhale.

Repeat four times.

Repeat standing on the right foot, and swing the left in a circle to the left.

Repeat, swinging each foot *backward* and around in a circle.

EXERCISE 95.—

Assume correct standing posture and inhale.

Poise the weight on the left foot and swing with the right foot, pointing the toes to the extreme right at the side, as far as you can reach.

Now swing the right leg forward in an arc, crossing over and touching the floor on the left side, as far as you can reach.

Exhale slowly, swinging back to the right.

Repeat four times.

Swing to position.

When you have become expert in balancing yourself, make the four swings rapidly while holding the breath.

Repeat, standing on the right foot, swinging the left.

EXERCISE 96.—Music, one-step. This exercise will limber the knees, strengthen the muscles of the legs and back and stimulate the circulation of the blood. It is also a good test for balance and rhythm.

(a) Assume the correct standing posture, hands on hips.

Inhale and hold.

Balancing the weight on the left, kick with the right leg from the *knee joint*. This will necessitate lifting the right leg (using the thigh muscles) a foot or more from the ground.

Kick four times, exhale slowly and resume position.

Repeat, balancing the weight on the right foot and kick with the left.

(b) Assume correct standing posture and inhale.

Balance the weight on the left foot and rise on the toes.

Lift the right foot and touch the ground about twelve inches in front.

Now kick from the *knee joint* and at the same time hop on the left foot, in time to the music. This will make two hops to each kick.

Repeat four times.

Resume position, exhaling slowly. Learn to control the timing of the breath and keep a regular rhythm.

Repeat with the left foot, hopping on the right.

Alternate, first kicking with the right foot and then with the left, in a rhythmic swinging motion.

(c) Repeat the above exercises, but kick from the *hip joint* and kick much higher. Kick four times with each foot.

Alternate, swinging the body in rhythmic motion, gracefully and lightly, with the action of the legs and feet.

EXERCISE 97.—Music, two-step or march. This exercise will strengthen and limber the knees and develop the muscles of the legs, back, and feet. It will also develop poise and balance.

Assume the correct standing posture, hands on hips.

Balance the weight on the left foot; inhale.

Lift the right knee to a level with the waist line and twirl the foot in a circle, from the knee joint. Whirl to the right four times.

Resume position and exhale slowly.

Repeat with the left leg, balancing on the right, four times.

EXERCISE 98.—Music, waltz or one-step. This exercise will employ nearly all the muscles of the body and will develop grace and poise at the same time.

(a) Assume the correct standing posture, hands at sides.

Balance the weight on the left leg and foot.

Inhale slowly while lifting the right arm forward in an arc, swinging it high above the head and backward, stretching vigorously all the way, with the fingers.

At the same time point the right foot forward, obliquely to the right, and stretch. This double movement will stretch all the muscles of the right side, promote the circulation of the blood and relieve obstructions of the nerves. Take it slowly and count six or nine.

Swing slowly to position, exhaling and counting three.

Repeat with the left arm, swinging the weight on to the right foot, stretching forward with the left.

(b) Repeat (a), but *twist* both the arm and the leg while extended. Twist first to the right and then to the left, vigorously and as far as you can, while stretching outward at the same time.

(c) Repeat (a) and (b) while stretching, but with the palm of the hand at the *wrist* instead of the fingers, thus bringing a different set of muscles under control.

(d) Repeat the motions as directed in (a), but stretch with the right hand and the *left* foot, keeping the balance of weight on the right.

Repeat, using the left hand and right foot.

Repeat (b) and (c) and alternate from one to the other to gain control and balance.

(e) Repeat all the exercises, stretching *forward* with the hands and *backward* with the feet.

Alternate forward and backward for control.

Exercise 99.—Music, any rhythmic tuneful melody in ¾ time.

(a) Assume correct standing posture; left hand on hip.

Poise the weight on the left foot and leg.

Inhale slowly and—

Swing the right arm forward, up and above the head and stretch all the way with the wrist leading and carry the hand back as far as you can and stretch up and back with the fingers, counting six or nine.

At the same time stretch forward with the right foot, obliquely to the right.

Now, turning the hand so that the palm of the wrist leads, swing the arm down toward the right foot, pulling all the way. A sweeping swing of the body and a graceful bending at the *hip joints,* and a slight spring at the knees (at first) will bring many muscles into play and assist wonderfully in establishing poise and balance. As the right hand nears the toes, reach forward gracefully and stretch with the fingers.

All of the movements should be done slowly and in perfect rhythm, counting nine and exhaling slowly on the downward bend.

Swing up again with a quicker motion, counting three, and stretching upward all the way.

Resume position. Count three.

Repeat four times with each hand, poising on the left foot when swinging the left arm, and placing the right hand on the hip.

(b) Alternate and accelerate the speed of all the motions to obtain rhythm and balance.

Exercise 100.—This exercise is excellent for limbering the hip and shoulder joints and for developing the muscles in the arms, legs, and back.

(a) Assume the correct standing posture, arms at sides.

Balance the weight on the left foot and leg.

Inhale slowly while placing the left hand on the left hip and, at the same time—

Lift the right arm forward in front on a level with the chest, counting three and, at the same time—

Place the right foot forward, obliquely to the right, pointing the toes.

Swing the right arm in a complete circle down and backward, up and around and with a sweeping bend at the hips (not the waist) bring the body forward and swing the hand around and down until you touch the toes. Count six. Exhale while bending.

Swing back to position, reversing the movement, swinging a circle with the arm and counting three. Inhale slowly and—

Resume position.

Repeat four times.

Repeat, with the left hand and left foot.

(b) Repeat, with the right hand and left foot.

Repeat, with the left hand and right foot.

(c) Repeat, standing with the feet apart and use both hands and swing the hands to the toes, being careful to bend at the hip joints rather than the waist.

(d) Repeat one exercise after the other in rapid succession to attain balance and quick control. This can be done only after much practice.

EXERCISE 101.—Music, one-step or march.

(a) Assume the correct standing posture, hands at sides, palms back.

Inhale and balance the weight on the left foot and leg. Count four.

Lift the right leg straight out in front, knee straight, as high as you can and keep your balance, stretching the heel forward and out.

Bend the left knee and sink the weight of the body slowly and steadily toward the floor until you touch the floor with your hands. (Touch the floor with the palms of the hands if able to without strain.) Count eight.

Assume standing posture, doing all the work possible with the left thigh and tendon Achilles. Be careful to keep the spine flexible. Count four.

(It may be necessary to steady yourself with the left hand on a chair, at first.) With proficiency it will soon be possible to perform the exercise without the use of any support and without touching the hands to the floor at all. At all times guard against flabby abdominal muscles, keep them well in and up.

Repeat with the other foot.

(b) Repeat exercise (a) with the arms folded. This will not be so difficult after you have mastered (a).

(c) Repeat exercise (b), alternating from one foot to the other with a slight spring as the change is made. This will develop great strength in the legs and back and splendid control.

This exercise may be done to dance music, and fast, as the Russian dancers do. Many variations may be added, such as turning, circling, twisting, and using the arms in a multitude of graceful ways.

Exercise 102.—Music, waltz time.

Assume correct standing posture, hands at sides.

Inhale, place hands on hips, balance the weight on the left foot and leg, counting three.

Bend the left knee and lower the body, keeping the right foot out in front, counting six.

Swing the right foot to the right and around back in an arc. Count six.

Bring foot to position, exhaling and—

Shift the weight to the right foot while placing the left foot out front, inhaling at the same time and counting six.

Repeat with the left foot, etc.

If necessary steady yourself by placing one hand on the seat of a chair until you gain sufficient strength to perform the exercise with the hands on the hips and, harder still, with the hands folded. Fine for poise.

Dancing Exercises

Exercise 103.—Music, one-step or two-step.

(a) Assume the correct standing posture, hands on hips.

Inhale rhythmically throughout the exercise.

Balance the weight on the ball of the left foot, rising forward on to the toes when dancing. Keep both knees and ankles limber.

Kick with the right foot in time to the music and hop on the left with each kick of the right.

With the toes pointed, kick forward, up, and outward about on a level with the waist. Increase the height of the kick with practice.

Each time the foot should be brought back to the floor, toes pointed and close to the left foot.

Repeat four times.

Repeat with the left foot kicking, hopping on the right.

(b) Repeat the movements of (a), but kick obliquely to the right, using the left foot to hop and the right foot to kick.

Repeat with the left foot kicking, hopping on the right.

(c) Now alternate, kicking first with the right and then with the left foot.

Repeat, kicking higher each time. Keep a rhythmic swing and a perfect balance.

EXERCISE 104.—Music, one-step or two-step.

(a) Assume correct standing posture, hands on hips.

Balance weight on left foot and leg. Inhale, counting three.

Lift right knee on a level with the waist, toes pointed down.

Kick from the knee joint, straight out in front. Count six.

Repeat three times without bringing the right foot to the floor. Keep poised on the ball of the left foot, springing with each kick.

Assume position, exhaling.

Repeat with the left foot, standing on the right.

(b) Repeat the movements of (a), but hop on the left foot with each kick of the right, and kick keeping the knee straight but not stiff.

Repeat with the right foot.

This is a good test for balance, especially if you kick first with the toes pointed and then with the heel, bringing a different set of muscles into play with each kick.

EXERCISE 105.—Music, ¾ time. This exercise brings the muscles of the back into play as well as the legs and develops control and balance.

(a) Assume the correct standing posture, hands on hips.

Balance the weight on the left foot and leg, being very careful not to allow the least tenseness in the hips, back, or legs during the movements, except those of stretching.

Inhale slowly and—

Lift the right leg up and out at the side as far as you can, stretching with the toes vigorously. Keep the knee straight but not rigid.

Repeat three times, holding the breath.

Resume position and exhale.

Repeat with the left foot.

Alternate, breathing rhythmically. Do not attempt to work too fast.

(b) Repeat (a) and stretch with the heels, vigorously, first with one foot and then with the other.

(c) Alternate, stretching first with the heels and then with the toes.

(d) Repeat exercises (a), (b), and (c), moving the legs straight back and out as far as you can. There is a greater tendency to stiffen the legs or buttocks with the backward stretch than with any other and bring undue pressure upon the spine with a constant jarring of the delicate nerves, thus affecting the entire nervous system.

(e) Repeat exercises (a), (b), and (c) with a swift and easy kick instead of the stretching. Then, leaning forward, repeat (d), kicking.

(f) Repeat (e) and alternate the forward kick with the back kick. Kick forward with the right foot and then with the left; then back with the right foot and then with the left; then forward with the right foot and then with the left, and so on.

(g) Kick to the right side and then to the left, alternating swiftly.

The Slave Walk

EXERCISE 106.—Music, an impressive march. This exercise is excellent for developing the muscles of the legs, back, and arms and for gaining control of the entire body. It is a splendid exercise and a test for balance and poise as well as rhythmic action. Unless done correctly, it is of little value.

(a) Assume the correct standing posture, hands at sides.

Inhale and clasp hands behind you, at the base of the spine. Count four.

At the same time place the weight on the left foot and leg and prepare to walk. All of the rules of posture and walking must be obeyed in this exercise. The breath should be rhyth-

mic, always holding it for the pull. Be very sure to hold t
abdominal muscles well in and up.

Taking a very long step with the right foot, swing the weig
of the body forward on to the right foot and thigh, wi
the right knee deeply bent. Balance with the toes of the l
foot. Count four. (Figure 42.)

Now *pull* with the forward swing with the shoulders, as thou
dragging a heavy weight. Count four.

When properly done the body will be swung well forward, t
trunk form a straight line with the left leg and the shoulde
be about on a line above the right knee. Be careful to ke
the feet straight ahead, the spine perfectly limber and t
hips, knees, and ankles flexible during all carrying and ba
ancing movements.

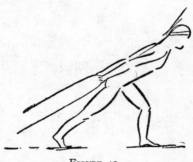

FIGURE 42

You will naturally exhale at the finish of the pull and the li
of the left foot forward for the next step. Count four.

Swing the left foot as far forward as you can for the ne
step, lifting the body up and forward as you swing ar
allowing the weight of the body to propel the forward motio
Repeat the pull with the shoulders.

(b) Repeat (a), except that the right hand should stretch forwar
as though reaching for some object when the weight
swung forward on to the right foot. The left hand shou
be poised on a line with the body to maintain balance. Vi
versa with the left hand.

(c) The leg movements and weight placement are practically tl
same in this exercise as for (b). With each step forwar

with the right foot reach forward with the right hand for an
imaginary object—out of reach, on the floor.

Repeat with the left hand, weight on the left foot, forward.
This is a good exercise for all the muscles of the body and
develops great body control and balance.

(d) Employ the same leg movements and weight placements in this
exercise as in (a).

Reach forward straight ahead of you with both hands as for an
imaginary object. Grasp firmly with the fists and pull back
with all your strength until your hands are as far back of
you as you can pull. At the same time you will push hard
with the left leg, straightened, and intensely pushing to brace
yourself, the weight poised on the right.

Repeat several times. This exercise is best practiced out-of-
doors; the beach, a garden or playground is ideal. The exercise may be intensified on an up or down grade.

EXERCISE 107.—The "slave walk" may be varied in a number of
teresting ways, such as reaching up and forward and dragging the
aginary object back toward the left or right, to the ground: turning
 pull from the rear on the forward step with both hands, first on
e side and then on the other. An interesting movement is to swing
e right arm back, up and around in a circle and throw an imaginary
ll forward, as you swing forward on to the right foot. Repeat with
e left, and so on. The double swing with both arms is more difficult.
 is interesting to try out experiments for yourself and develop new
ercises. But remember always to keep within the laws of correct pos-
re, carriage, and balance, with flexible spine and joints.

he Indian System Applied to Work

Everyone, while at his vocation or at play, can develop his body
 the same time. A little thought and effort will form new habits,
orking both automatically. With habits once formed it would seem
resome and awkward to do any other way.

There is a right way and a wrong way to do everything. The Indian
nsiders that time and energy are too precious to be wasted, so he
ncentrates his efforts, mentally and physically, by employing the
me system of body development and weight placement in his labor
at he uses in his exercise or games.

And so, with manual labor, put your thoughts and will power into it, as the Indian does, making it accomplish a double purpose: over coming old habits and rebuilding the body at the same time. Get th joy out of work by doing both the work and the exercise as well as yo possibly can. And do not be too easily satisfied—strive rather for pe fection—there is always something more to learn. As we reach pe fection in one line we have the opportunity of teaching others, passin the good work along, and soon a way opens for still greater achiev ment—automatically brought about by the law of cause and effect— a compensation.

The western cowboy has absorbed much of the Indian's athleti psychology in his years of contact with the red man and has adapte many of the Indian's methods to his own use. With his daring spir and quick wit he has added a surprising number of stunts and dare-dev feats which make him an athlete to be reckoned with and in a clas quite by himself. Whether breaking a broncho or merely handling pail of water, he applies the same basic methods and—*thinks while h does it*. He thinks and *wills* strength into his body. Accuracy an efficiency together with lightning speed accompany his actions, coolnes and absolute self-control dominate his emotions and calm, fearles decision occupies his mind.

There are many forms of labor extremely useful in physical devel opment, such as digging, gardening, chopping wood, pitching hay pruning trees and many outdoor jobs, such as cleaning automobiles keeping up the lawn, etc. There is no better all-round exercise fo women than housework. Sweeping, cleaning, kneading bread, an even dish-washing may be made a valuable exercise by introducing th right movements while working. Breathe rhythmically, stand correctly place the weight where it belongs, use the arms and hands gracefully poise the head carefully, use the eyes accurately—and above all—*thin right*. Plans for the systematic management of the home, the meals, th children—all may be worked out mentally while disposing of the dishes Great problems of love, happiness, unselfishness, and sacrifice hav been solved over the dish pan!

Simplified living would reduce the cost of living and preserve th health of the family as well, to say nothing of conquering half th drudgery. Far too much time and energy are wasted over fancy dishe and elaborate meals, catering to abnormal appetites, desires and greed— labor which only causes sickness, expense and more labor later— nursing and doctor bills. Simplicity is the keynote to health an longevity. It might be wise to follow the Indian's philosophy of life and develop an appreciation for the values hidden in the common things of life.

When reaching, lifting, pulling, or shoving, follow the rules of weight placement and posture, and apply the exercises given herein. Let the big muscles do the major part. Experiment, study yourself and your body, and learn to do your work scientifically, using the least amount of energy to accomplish the greatest amount of work. Let your head save your energy. Think before you act and then think with the action.

Reaching

EXERCISE 108.—When reaching for small or medium-sized objects be careful to follow the rules for posture and weight placement. Reaching is good exercise when properly done; habits formed while reaching for the lesser things will work spontaneously when reaching for large or heavy objects where real strength and head-work are required.

Get a good firm stance with the feet wide enough apart to feel secure, and do the major part of the balancing with the thighs to carry the weight. A very heavy weight cannot be handled with the feet close together.

Take a deep breath, brace the diaphragm and the abdominal muscles firmly, in and up, to keep the vital organs in place, and be sure to work with a flexible spine; you will have twice the power and will be much better able to maintain perfect balance.

Stretch the muscles of the arms, legs, and joints and learn to balance the body without any means of support or without leaning against anything.

In ordinary reaching for comparatively small objects on shelves, the weight is usually placed over the foot and leg on the same side as the arm used. Keep the other hand ready to assist—always on the alert.

Method

Assume correct standing posture.

Inhale and place weight on right foot and leg.

Sway slightly forward as you reach upward with the right hand, allowing the wrist to lead the movement. Use both hands if the object is heavy. Never attempt to reach for any object with one hand in your pocket or on the hip; keep it in readiness to balance the object reached for or to assist in case of accident, either to grasp the object or hold your balance.

Grasp the object firmly, rising on the toes if necessary to get a good hold, then, holding the breath. (Figure 43)

Lower the heels to the floor, using the muscles of the arms, shoulders and hands, and bring the object to any desired position.

Exhale and relax to position.

Do not do all of your work with the right hand. Try to use the left as often as you do the right hand. Train the left hand and arm to become as actively useful as the right; this will insure an even develop-

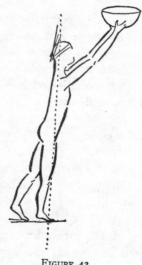

FIGURE 43

ment of the muscles and will help you to acquire greater poise and balance as well as add to your efficiency, physically and mentally. To use the left hand and arm necessitates using the eye, the mind and the brain as well as the muscles and nerves on the other side of your body. Become ambidextrous, so that in case of accident to either member you will not be so hampered—it is all a matter of culture and self-training.

EXERCISE 109.—In preparing to lift a heavy object it is advisable to take three deep breaths and concentrate upon vitalizing the body. It is necessary also to have perfect confidence that you can successfully lift the object without dropping it and without injury to yourself. If you know that the weight is beyond your strength and that you might run the risk of overstrain, do not attempt it. It is better to train the muscles gradually to carry any desired load. The effect of overstraining is bad upon the heart as well as the lungs and nerves; the danger of accident is oftentimes very serious. An attempt to "show off" or "take a dare" may injure you for life—it is very foolish. Use common sense and do not be "bullied" into attempts beyond your strength.

Follow the rules for posture and weight placement, being careful to keep the spine flexible.

Get a firm stance with the feet wide enough apart to form an arch of the legs. (The arch is the strongest form of architecture known.)

Bend the knees, keeping the weight placed well upon the thighs and poised over the arches of the feet, allowing the tendon Achilles at the back of the heel to act with the thigh as double leverage, using the knees and ankles as fulcrums.

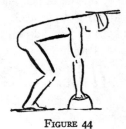

FIGURE 44

Grasp the object to be lifted firmly with both hands.

Take a deep breath and hold, bracing the diaphragm and the abdominal muscles firmly in and up to hold the viscera in place and act as a protection against sudden strain or rupture.

Do not attempt to lift the hands alone but, holding the object firmly, lift your entire body by the muscles of the legs. This will throw the work on the largest and strongest muscles of the body and prevent any undue strain upon the spine or the small of the back. The muscles of the arms, shoulders, sides, and back will naturally assume their proper share of the burden. The back will arch somewhat—quite naturally. (Figure 44.)

Whether the burden is to be raised to a higher level, moved to the side, or the front, or carried, the same rules apply. The arms, hands, and shoulders act much as a crane does—the power for the weight and propulsion are in the machinery of the legs.

Exhale slowly when the burden is deposited, or, if it is to be carried, breath rhythmically and principally in the upper portions of the lungs, holding the abdominal walls firmly in and up.

Power Lifting

EXERCISE 110.—By going through the motions as described above and lifting an imaginary weight, great strength and ability may be acquired.

Similar development may be obtained by practicing the following instructions for pushing and pulling, but with an imaginary heavy weight or force, and by positively directing the will power.

Get a firm stance with the feet wide apart; inhale and hold. Count four. Be careful to observe the rules of posture and abdominal muscular control.

Bend the knees and lower the body, balancing forward, and do all the work with the legs, keeping the hands and arms relaxed, allowing them to fall forward toward the object to be lifted.

Grasp the object with both hands and pull up with all your strength with the legs until you stand straight, then lift with the arms, using the large muscles until the imaginary weight is above the head, and then push. Feel the pull and effort in the muscles from the finger tips to the toes. Additional effort may be used by bringing the feet together, rising on the toes and pushing still higher.

Exhale slowly as you resume correct standing posture. Breathe three times rhythmically before repeating the exercise.

Shoving or Pushing

EXERCISE 111.—The rules for posture and weight placement are the same for shoving and pushing as for lifting. Brace the feet firmly, gripping the ground with the feet for support; use the legs for power.

The shoulders, arms and hands act as secondary means of propulsion. The muscles of the back form an arch or bridge between the action of the legs and arms. Be careful not to let the small of the back curve in too much and thereby take the brunt of the weight at a wrong angle. This often causes strain or rupture.

Assume the correct standing posture in front of the object to be shoved.

Inhale deeply as you place one foot a little ahead of the other and place your hands conveniently against the object as near the region of the shoulders as possible, as it is here the best leverage is maintained.

Grip the ground firmly with the feet and use the muscles of the legs to do the principal part of the work. Even when walking, while shoving a heavy object, the main part of the work can be done with the legs. (Figure 45.)

It is better to rest and exhale slowly than to attempt breathing while shoving with the full extent of your strength. Then take another deep breath and proceed.

The Indians respect a certain rhythm in all their heavy lifting, pushing, and pulling, working in unison and timing the rhythm to the breath. Sailors work in a similar fashion, sometimes singing a monosyl-

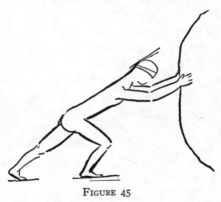

FIGURE 45

labic melody for encouragement or confidence and to facilitate working together in accurately timed efforts.

Pulling

EXERCISE 112.—The rules for posture and weight placement are the same for pulling as for lifting. Get a good firm stance, spread the feet slightly, a foot or so apart, distribute the weight evenly and emphasize the stance with the thighs as well.

Take a deep breath while reaching for the object and hold.

Grasp the object firmly with both hands and pull, easily at first, to gauge the amount of strength needed, then steadily as you become accustomed to the weight. The muscles of the shoulders, arms and hands serve to hold and the muscles of the legs do the principal part of the work—the back acting as a bridge.

Exhale and breathe deeply before the next pull.

Always concentrate the will upon accomplishing the task—and with certainty of success. Learn to have perfect confidence in yourself —confidence based on past performance and a knowledge of your ability and confidence in that supreme All Power acting through you.

If pulling a heavy object while moving, whether walking backward or forward, always allow the legs to assume the heaviest part of the burden. (Figure 42.)

When pulling up from the ground, directly or vertically, the position should be practically the same as for lifting and the principal burden assumed by the legs.

It is particularly important to keep the spine flexible when moving heavy objects. It is then easier to maintain a perfect balance without injury and facilitates quick movement in any direction. Further, there is less jar upon the super-sensitive nerves of the spine, especially in case of accident, falling or slipping.

In pulling an imaginary object from above, concentrate the will upon attaining a tremendous vital power which you wish to draw through your body for *good* use.

Ground Work

When performing any kind of work close to the ground it is advisable to practice the various forms of squatting and kneeling. The spine should be flexible and the weight placed upon the legs. Keep the knees limber with exercises so that you will not feel the strain when working.

EXERCISE 113.—Assume the correct standing posture and inhale.

With the weight poised slightly forward, lower the body toward the ground, bending the knees and ankles as the thighs take the burden of the weight and the tendons Achilles guide and support the motion. Hold the breath during the descent.

The lower you squat the more the weight is naturally thrown forward so that a rise on to the balls of the feet is necessary and comfortable.

If you work with the hands straight in front it may be necessary to spread the knees. If at the side, your knees will naturally swing a little in the opposite direction. It is restful to change about. The Indian is so in the habit of squatting and even moving about in that position that he seldom tires. Anyone can do it—it is merely a matter of practice.

If you intend rising immediately, hold the breath while accomplishing the act and exhale upon rising. If you remain squatting for any length of time, breathe rhythmically.

Indians do much of their ground work on their knees, sometimes resting back upon the heels and sometimes propelling their movements to the right or left and backward or forward. The principle remains the same—the work is done mainly with the thighs, the spine remaining flexible and sometimes relaxed. The arms and hands should accomplish their work from the shoulder joint. (Figures 29 and 31.)

The cross-legged sitting position is almost as popular with Indians as kneeling or squatting for they like to be in contact with Mother Earth while working and enjoy the benefits of her electric and magnetic currents which are believed to pass through their bodies. (Figure 30.)

In any of these positions the Indian is taught not to slouch but to hold himself with becoming dignity, obeying the rules of correct sitting posture with all sense organs quietly alert. Sleepy looking Indians seldom miss anything that is going on about them—they are silently observant, weighing and considering with keen interest but with controlled thoughts.